GET YOUR FAMILY EATING RIGHT!

A 30-Day Plan for Teaching Your Kids Healthy Eating Habits for Life

LYNN FREDERICKS
Founder, Family Cook Productions

MERCEDES SANCHEZ,
M.S., R.D.
Director of Nutrition Education,
Family Cook Productions

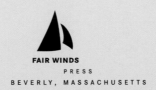

FAIR WINDS
PRESS
BEVERLY, MASSACHUSETTS

First published in the USA in 2013 by
Fair Winds Press, a member of
Quayside Publishing Group
100 Cummings Center
Suite 406-L
Beverly, MA 01915-6101
www.fairwindspress.com

17 16 15 14 13 1 2 3 4 5

ISBN: 978-1-59233-550-3

Digital edition published in 2013
eISBN: 978-1-61058-745-7

Library of Congress Cataloging-in-Publication Data available

Cover and book design by Debbie Berne
Photography by Glenn Scott Photography
Food styling by Alisa Neely
Shutterstock.com: pages 8, 16, 30, 38, 60, 73, 83, 90, 108, 128,
166, 186, 194

Printed and bound in China

The information in this book is for educational purposes only.
It is not intended to replace the advice of a physician or medical
practitioner. Please see your health care provider before beginning any new health program.

Lynn: to Alex, Stephan and my dear mother and grandmother, Eileen and Ann.

♡

Merche: to Bruno, Sofia, David and my mother. Antonia.

♡

contents

Introduction

ARE YOU READY to turn the tables on the way your family eats? Then you've come to the right place. If you bought this book, you probably take your role as the provider of your family's meals seriously. And because we understand that role is challenging, we'd like to offer some easy-to-digest guidance and creative ways to make the process fun. We are delighted to share with you strategies to help your family eat both healthfully and joyfully each day—for life.

We are mothers who have experienced our own family food challenges. At FamilyCook Productions, we use our experiences—along with our professional knowledge and our passion for family meals—to create educational programming that has had a positive impact on more than 100,000 families around the world.

Our curricula promote plant-based recipes that use fruits, vegetables, grains, seeds, and nuts. We take a multicultural approach, choosing recipes from many lands and exploring the relationships different cultures have with food. We inspire children to eat healthy foods by engaging them in an all-sensory cooking experience. Every lesson involves an abundance of aromas, colors, textures, tastes, and sounds to encourage kids to be adventurous and try new foods. We strive to create a festive, memorable experience for everyone—our FamilyCook classrooms are experiential learning laboratories.

Since 1998, we have worked together, honing our best strategies and discarding tactics that did not work in the family setting. In this book, we share our most successful approaches with you.

lynn fredericks's experience

I invited my children to cook our meals with me when I was a newly divorced mother of two young boys—one a toddler. Bonding around the creative activity of cooking helped my sons and me heal from the divorce. Over the years, my family life improved dramatically as we shared quality time together, making recipes from around the world.

By the time my younger son, Stephan, was seven, seafood risotto had become his specialty. His adolescent brother developed into an amazing sous chef. Laughter and smiles filled our kitchen, and the pressure of single parenthood eased a bit each evening as we prepared and shared a delicious, healthy meal together. Now in their twenties and living independently, my children cook for themselves—Stephan even makes his own bread.

I learned so much about cooking with children that I wanted to share this wisdom with other families. I shifted from being a food writer for magazines and newspapers to being an educator. I took the secrets I'd learned from chefs of various cuisines—American, French, Italian, and Asian in particular—and pared them down to the essentials, so I could teach parents how to cook with their children at home. In 1995, I founded what would become FamilyCook Productions and later wrote my first book *Cooking Time Is Family Time*.

We now work with partners from New York to Brazil, employing our field-tested, evidence-based strategies and our specific philosophy. We show people how to make healthier choices, first and foremost by inspiring enjoyment. HealthCorps, founded by surgeon and health expert Dr. Oz, licensed our "Teen Battle Chef" program to schools across the United States. The American Heart Association and Dole/Tropicana juices support our preschool program, "Nibble 1, 2, 3 with Willow." Together, we are successfully moving parents and children toward a healthier relationship with food.

mercedes sanchez's experience

For me, food offered a way to connect my children with their Spanish origins. The birth of my first child prompted me to reflect on who I was, so I could explain our heritage to my daughter, Sofia. Although I'd left Spain in my twenties to settle in the United States, it was not until I became a new mother that I began to feel like the immigrant I was.

In a country where few people knew much about Spain, I searched for foods and recipes from my homeland. With each Spanish meal I served, I regaled Sofia with the stories behind every recipe. In this way, I connected my daughter with my Spanish family and origins.

My French-American husband also began to search for his roots and voilà, a new pride for French cuisine emerged. Surprisingly, our newfound interest in our different heritages created an obstacle. We debated which was better, manchego cheese or brie? Spanish jamón or foie gras? One of our biggest battles centered on whether to fry an egg with olive oil or butter. Would eggs become grounds for divorce?

Despite such challenges, I persevered and insisted that my children literally consume their Spanish and French heritages. Thanks to my work with Lynn, we happily adopted the culinary diversity of America into our family diet.

After I became a registered dietician, I also focused on the nutritional value of our meals. I endeavored to serve mostly whole foods and struggled to limit unhealthy ones. My most successful tactics have been shared through FamilyCook Productions' program for more than fifteen years. In this book, I am excited to share them with you.

how this book can help your family

Our philosophy has four essential objectives emphasized throughout this book:

1. Enjoy meals at the table together.
2. Eat meals cooked at home.
3. Cook with fresh ingredients.
4. Let everyone help.

Sound easy? Well, we're not going to lie to you—it will take some effort. But we do have lots of tricks up our sleeves to share with you to make it fun and, above all, easier. We'll show you how to feed your family delicious, simple, healthy meals and save money, too.

Eating Healthy Meals Can Be a Pleasurable Experience

Eating is a social act, and children learn to eat healthy foods through sharing home-cooked meals with family and friends. In this way, children associate real food first with a pleasurable experience and, by default, learn that it's good for them.

A healthy, balanced diet means eating a variety of whole, fresh, and minimally processed foods from all the food groups. We give special attention to seasonal fruits and vegetables, whole grains, and plant-based foods. This diet is naturally low in fat and rich in essential nutrients, and thereby it helps children and adults to maintain healthy weights.

Cooking healthy foods that taste delicious does not have to be complicated or time consuming. In this book, we provide global strategies and recipes that offer American tables a welcome and exciting change.

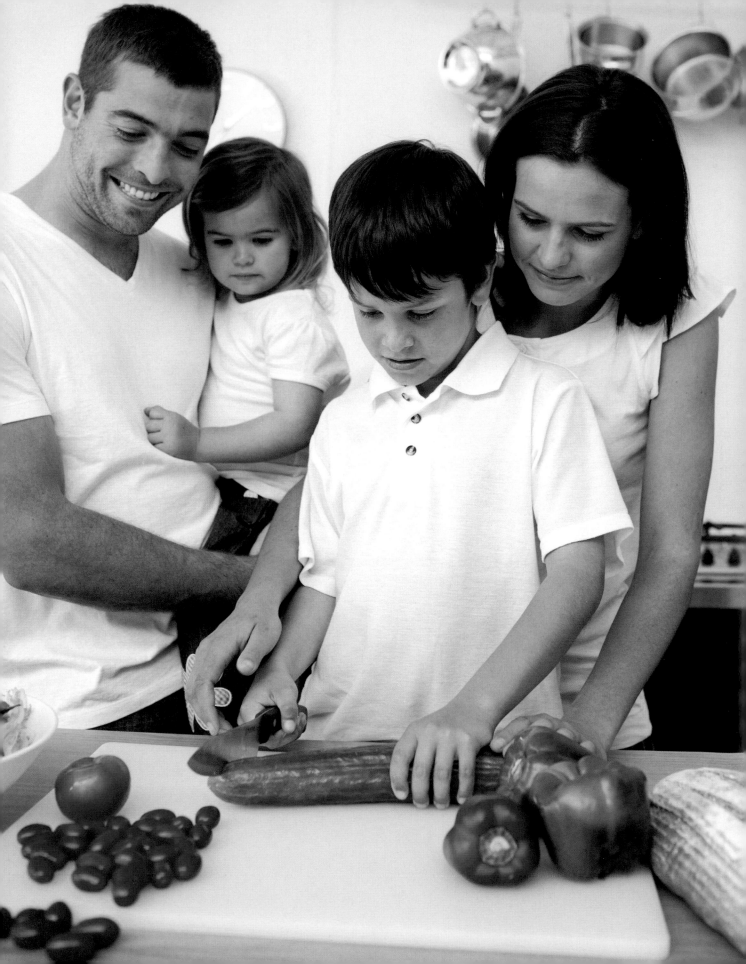

Get Kids to Try New Foods by Giving Them a Sensory Experience

Inviting children to cook is the best way to introduce them to new foods. Cooking and tasting engage all their senses. As children cut, squeeze, and press fresh ingredients, and use herbs and spices in preparing a dish, they enjoy the fragrances. They feel textures with surprise. They admire the colors. This multisensory exposure encourages children to taste the final product—vegetables and all.

We use multicultural themes to teach the importance of food in every culture, including our own. So be prepared: In addition to changing how you eat, we are going to spice up your family meals with some international flavors. Our message is to pay attention to what you eat, select local ingredients, and celebrate the season—and we reinforce it in a fun, memorable way. Not surprisingly, these positive associations build enthusiasm in parents and children and make it easier to start cooking at home as a family.

What You'll Learn from This Book

Through preparing the simple and delicious recipes we share, you and your children will develop the following:

- ♡ basic cooking skills
- ♡ nutrition fundamentals
- ♡ an adventurous nature when it comes to trying new foods
- ♡ an interest in sharing meals at the table with family and friends
- ♡ more cultural awareness and tolerance

How do you begin? Start with our first step on Day 1. Here we outline issues you need to think about to get the most from this book. Each day in our

We know it takes a shift in values and mindset—changing your attitudes about meal planning and cooking—before real change can take place.

thirty-day plan follows an intentional sequence. It may not seem exactly intuitive—for instance, cooking skills don't come in until Day 11. But in our eighteen-plus years of working with thousands of families, we know it takes a shift in values and mindset—changing your attitudes about meal planning and cooking—before real change can take place. Only then do we provide readers with culinary fundamentals, particularly knife techniques, to instill skills and confidence.

When you feel confident with your new skills and realize that preparing recipes with lots of fresh vegetables is not too much work, you're ready to bring your children in to help. We'll show you how to create a foundation for cooking delicious, simple recipes together. You'll embark on a culinary journey around the world, making and enjoying colorful, flavorful, and healthy meals as a family. The recipes become a bit more ambitious as you go along, so you can skip ahead if you are already a confident cook. Otherwise, we recommend you follow the steps in sequence. Above all, progress at your own pace.

In most chapters you will find recipes that provide tasty opportunities to try out new strategies for preparing meals with your children. We're confident your family will find many delicious favorites to make over and over again.

PART 1

GETTING STARTED

{ DAY 1 } Embrace Change

THIS FIRST STEP IS ABOUT YOU. You are beginning a new relationship with food. You are refocusing on the pleasure of eating and the joy it can bring you. Embrace the change. Take a deep breath, pour your favorite drink, sit down, relax, and clear your mind. Now visualize a pair of virtual kitchen shears, and snip away at the tangle of nutritional messages, dietary advice, picky eaters' preferences, calorie anxieties, and all the unpleasant memories you have about food preparation. Feeding a family can be daunting, time consuming, and frequently, unappreciated. You are going to remove these fears from your relationship with food.

What will it take to get there?

Why does a Japanese woman wake at 5:00 a.m. to buy freshly caught *toro*, the best and most tender part of tuna sushi, at the central market in downtown Tokyo? Why does an Italian search various markets for the best *pomodoro* ("tomato") and the freshest mozzarella cheese for his Caprese salad? Why might an Arab wait in long lines to eat the best hummus in town? Why did Lynn's father insist on going to one particular farm stand in her Illinois town for the freshest summer sweet corn? These people have found joy in everyday culinary pleasures and celebrate the food that is unique to their cultures.

get more pleasure from real food

Pause and ask yourself what *real* foods do you enjoy eating? What real foods hold pleasurable associations for you? Which taste good and give you a sense of

> **MISSION FOR THE DAY**
>
> Prepare your mind and kitchen for a new way of eating.

identity? Search within the culture you come from, and recall your favorite relative's recipes.

Make it a priority to find the best quality foods you can afford. Search farmers' markets for food that has been just harvested at its peak for ripeness and flavor. Fall in love with food. Give yourself time for the search and allow the love affair to develop.

Make eating special. Take your children to the right restaurants, or to stores where you can share with them your interest in good, affordable food.

Above all else, prepare the foods you love. Serve them and eat them with lust. Your children learn from watching you. We cannot tell you how many foods our children would not touch until watching us enjoy those foods piqued their interest.

get more enjoyment from your kitchen

As part of your new relationship with food, you are going to be spending more time in the kitchen, so let's take a new look at this room. Is your kitchen a space you enjoy? Or, is it dark, messy, or otherwise uninviting?

What simple changes could you make to enhance your enjoyment of your kitchen? Do you need brighter lights? Would live plants make it more appealing? How about music: Can you add a radio or mp3 player? Give your kitchen some TLC to create a comfortable and inviting space.

survey: which of our four objectives will be more challenging for you?				
behavior	rarely	sometimes	often	notes
enjoy meals at the table together				
eat meals cooked at home (not reheated)				
cook with fresh ingredients (minimal prepackaged food)				
let everyone help (spouse and children helping regularly)				

Are your kitchen's counters and surfaces free and uncluttered? If not, clear the clutter and free up space for cooking.

Zero in on any broken appliances or equipment that doesn't work (e.g., old toaster, busted blender). Repair, replace, or throw them out. Clean out your kitchen drawers and discard anything that is broken or rusty. Remove utility items: keep your drawers for cooking utensils. Add a drawer organizer so you can quickly find the tools you need.

Inspect your cupboards and fridge and purge them of items that have been there more than six months—unless you find a fabulous whole-grain pilaf that you haven't yet had time to prepare.

identify areas for improvement to help you meet your goals

Once you have prepared yourself internally (with a new attitude) and externally (with a cheerful and user-friendly kitchen), you're ready to begin an exciting journey. As you start, keep in mind the four objectives we identified in the introduction:

1. Enjoy meals at the table together.
2. Eat meals cooked at home.
3. Cook with fresh ingredients.
4. Let everyone help.

How often do you currently adhere to these four objectives? Use the chart above to assess where your family is right now, so you know where to focus your attention. It will help you to determine which of these objectives will be more challenging for you as you embark on our thirty-day plan.

What did this chart reveal? Let's analyze your responses.

Mostly "Rarely"
You have your work cut out for you. To make the change more manageable, focus on Objectives 1 and

reboot your mindset for success

Copy this list or flag it in your digital book, so you can refer to it anytime in the process when you become discouraged:

- Replace anxiety and fear of failure with resolve.
- Acknowledge that investing some time is necessary.
- Trust that persistence pays off.
- Commit to your goals despite setbacks.
- When you feel you've gotten off track (this is normal), reboot your mindset and start again.

2. Even if you don't cook everything from scratch with raw ingredients and take lots of short cuts, you will still make huge strides.

Mostly "Sometimes"

This book will help you advance from "well intentioned" to achieving most of the objectives with frequency. Our time-management tricks and guides on seasonal cooking will give you the confidence to easily practice all four objectives most of the time.

Mostly "Often"

You are doing everything right, so our book will get you to the next level. You'll enhance your knowledge and confidence, and maximize the nutritional value of all the meals you serve. You'll also learn some delicious new recipes and family cooking strategies.

Go on to the next step *only when you are ready.* We advise going out of sequence only if you are a skilled cook already and are mostly looking for healthy recipes and nutritional support. From our long experience, we know that changing the way your family eats requires being gentle yet firm with yourself as you commit to doing a little more each day. That's how this book works. Each day we coach you to the next step, so you enjoy the process and don't get overwhelmed. In just thirty days, you'll be making easy, delicious home-cooked meals that provide better nutrition—and you'll save money to boot!

{ DAY 2 } Make Family Meals a Priority

FOOD HAS A SPECIAL MEANING when it's shared, appreciated, and valued. People around the world have been eating together for millennia, sharing not only food but traditions and lore. In the process, they forge a cultural identity. Eating together offers an opportunity to reconnect with each other. Our ancestors also understood the significance of agriculture to their survival. Hence, harvest time was anticipated, appreciated, and celebrated with great fanfare. Although contemporary families may not have that immediate connection to the land, we can still appreciate and celebrate the food we eat. Children learn to eat traditional foods—chile peppers in Mexico, raw fish in Japan, fried ants in Cambodia—by imitating their parents' behaviors during shared meals. Whether those behaviors are healthy or unhealthy, they teach children eating habits for life. The choice is yours. What do you want to model for your children?

prioritize sit-down family meals to improve health and well-being

This may be one of the most important changes you can make toward creating a healthy family. Scientific studies show that when families sit down together for meals they eat more fruit and vegetables, less junk food, and enjoy better psycho-social health. According to the National Center on Addiction and Substance Abuse at Columbia University, eating together as a family improves children's grades in

school, increases self-esteem, and reduces the incidence of substance abuse.

Family dinners cooked at home are challenging for overscheduled families. However, the benefits of sharing meals justify the effort and give you an incentive to find the time. It's a matter of priorities, just like finding time to teach your children hygiene, the alphabet, or numbers.

establish mealtime rituals to bond as a family

Each culture has developed its own mealtime rituals and etiquette—saying a prayer or a word of thanks before a meal, waiting to eat until everyone has been served, or dressing for dinner. These rituals bring intention and meaning to the experience of eating. They provide a moment to pause and connect with one another, to refrain from gulping the food thoughtlessly, and to anticipate and appreciate the meal. When we eat a meal mindlessly on the go, we lose the meaning of what we eat, and it doesn't teach our children to appreciate our efforts.

In our school program, we teach children that harmony, respect, silence, and aesthetics are concepts appreciated in the Japanese tea ceremony.

When we eat a meal mindlessly on the go, we lose the meaning of what we eat, and it doesn't teach our children to appreciate our efforts.

We recreate the ceremony together. The children get so involved in the ritual that they end up drinking the bitter green tea. Everybody enjoys pronouncing *itadakimasu*, an ancient Japanese word still used today to acknowledge the beginning of something important, such as a meal.

set parameters to gain your family's cooperation

Your status as the person who satisfies everyone's hunger and provides the pleasure of delicious food is an inherently powerful platform. Use this platform with grace and confidence. Explain that it's your job to select the best ingredients and prepare nutritious meals, and you expect everyone to sit and enjoy meals together. In this way, you elevate your family's expectations about food and communicate your values.

Of course you may get some push back. But as you shrug off children's protests with firm messages about the food you serve, you establish parameters that, if you are consistent, will be accepted over time. It takes courage to stir things up in the family and face resistance as you work toward your goal. It takes effort and commitment. But the rewards are so great you'll have no regrets.

lynn's story

My family meal journey came full circle when I communicated to my children that enjoying our meal together at the table was as important as cooking it together. I declared our dining table a "sacred space" and banned toys, mail, and clutter from it. Our table was laid with an inexpensive, washable tablecloth and napkins in napkin rings. Everyone had a designated seat and used that same napkin until it was laundry day. I purchased an economy bag of tea lights, so the boys could light votive candles each evening. My message was clear:

- Dinnertime is a daily celebration we share over our delicious home-cooked meal.
- I will sit with you and give you all my attention while we are together at our table.

Making our meals a celebratory experience knit my family into a cohesive unit. Over time, this helped establish a strong family identity, deep appreciation, and love.

As someone who intentionally shifted my own values to make family meals a major focus of my family life, I can attest to the lasting benefits. The healthy communication my sons and I established during our family meals served us well during their challenging adolescent years. Now in their twenties, my sons are great cooks who are conscientious about the quality of the food they eat. They've also adopted the values I modeled about the importance of family meals. They consider the meals I prepare a supreme act of love and nurturing. To my delight, they usually prefer cooking and eating together at home rather than going out.

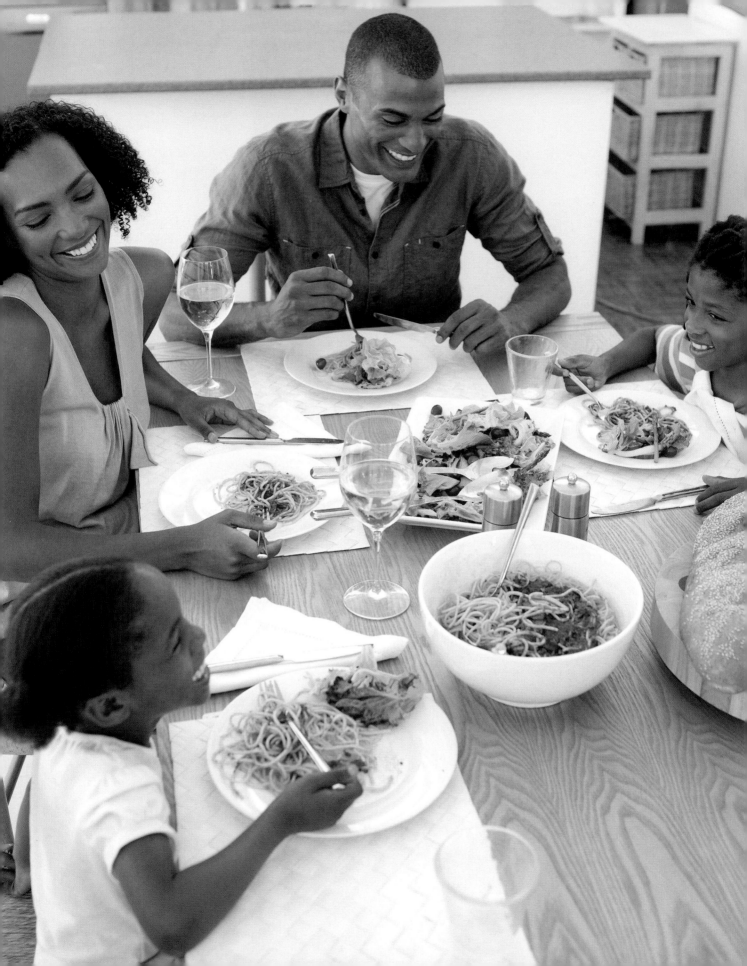

nine ways to make cooking time family time

1 Turn off the television at mealtime.

2 Share responsibility with your children for all aspects of the meal.

3 Shop for dinner with your children, giving them an opportunity to suggest new foods.

4 Establish your food budget and show children how cooking from scratch is more economical than using prepared foods.

5 Start with recipes they love; explain that if they want to eat it, they have to help make it.

6 Begin by asking an apathetic eater to help with a simple fruit dessert.

7 Make the dinner table sacred.

8 Wait until all family members are seated and served before anyone is permitted to begin eating.

9 Make it clear that during cooking time you're only available in the kitchen. If they need you, they are welcome to join you there.

get started

Remember this phrase whenever you get discouraged. Think of it as your mantra: "*Your family meals are sacred and nourish your family in mind, body, and spirit.*" Here are some ways to help you put this mantra into practice:

♡ Consider your family's schedule. How can you extend a sit-down family meal so it isn't rushed? How about a brunch on the weekend?

♡ Prolong meals for a few minutes so all family members can share their news of the day.

♡ Establish a ritual for your family meals. Come up with a few ideas and let your family choose.

♡ Delegate responsibilities. Make a chart that states who sets or clears the table or cleans pots and on which days. Make sure everyone agrees; that way it's easier to remind them, and you leave less space for negotiation.

Your status as the person who satisfies everyone's hunger and provides the pleasure of delicious food is an inherently powerful platform.

three sisters salad

This easy recipe is a hit with children because using the shredding tool is super fun and magical. The combination of corn and tomatoes with lemon gives a tangy-sweet result.

1 medium zucchini

1 ear sweet corn, or 1 can (15 ounces, or 430 g) corn, drained

1 can (15 ounces, or 430 g) white cannellini beans, drained and rinsed

15 grape or cherry tomatoes

5 sprigs fresh basil

2 tablespoons (30 ml) olive oil

1 lemon

Salt and pepper

SPECIAL EQUIPMENT
Asian shredding tool (available at Asian markets and online) or grater

NOTE: *Children should use plastic or table knives for all child steps that require cutting or chopping.*

ADULT & CHILD Shred the zucchini using a shredding tool or a grater, using the setting for the largest-size pieces. Place shredded zucchini in a large mixing bowl.

ADULT Slice the bottom of the corn off the cob, and stand on the flat bottom. Slice the kernels off the fresh ears of corn and add to the bowl.

CHILD Add the drained beans to the bowl. Mix well.

ADULT & CHILD Slice the tomatoes in half using a table knife. Add to bowl.

ADULT & CHILD Remove the basil leaves from the stems. Chop the leaves and add to the bowl.

ADULT & CHILD Measure and add the olive oil. Squeeze the lemon over the bowl and mix well. Season to taste with salt and pepper, and serve.

PREP TIME	YIELD
15 minutes	6 to 8 servings

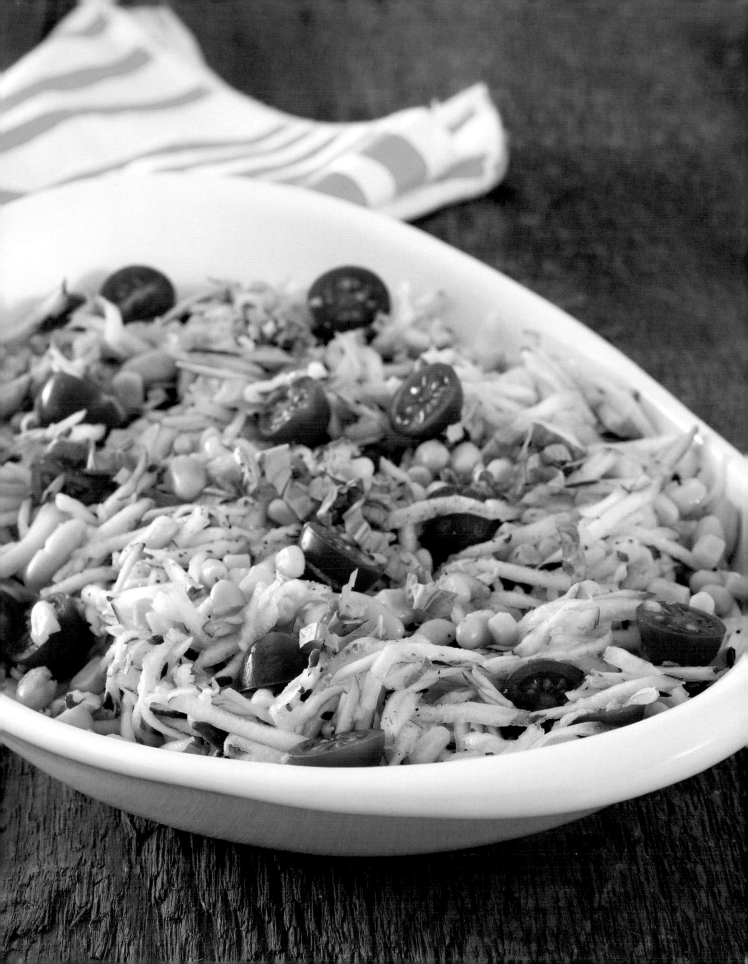

chocolate fondue with fruit

Here's a terrific opportunity to enjoy seasonal fruit or the diversity of tropical fruit. Try to include all the colors of the spectrum. It's a great way to get your kids to sample something new.

½ pound (225g) semisweet or milk chocolate

2 pounds (907 g) fresh seasonal fruit, in a variety of colors

NOTE: *Children should use plastic or table knives for all child steps that require cutting or chopping.*

ADULT Place the chocolate in a microwavable bowl, not plastic, and melt in the microwave on High for 1 minute. Remove and stir. If necessary, repeat for 30 seconds at a time, until the chocolate is smooth.

ADULT & CHILD While the chocolate is melting, the adult can slice, core, or pit the seasonal fruit. Children can help cut pieces in half or slice the fruit into bite-size pieces for dipping.

CHILD Arrange the fruit pieces on plates in a fun design.

ADULT Transfer melted chocolate to a small bowl for dipping.

ADULT & CHILD Each family member can dip a piece of fruit by hand or fork directly into the warm chocolate.

OPTIONAL: Place a dollop of warm chocolate on each individual plate.

PREP TIME	COOK TIME	YIELD
10 minutes	1 to 3 minutes	4 to 6 servings

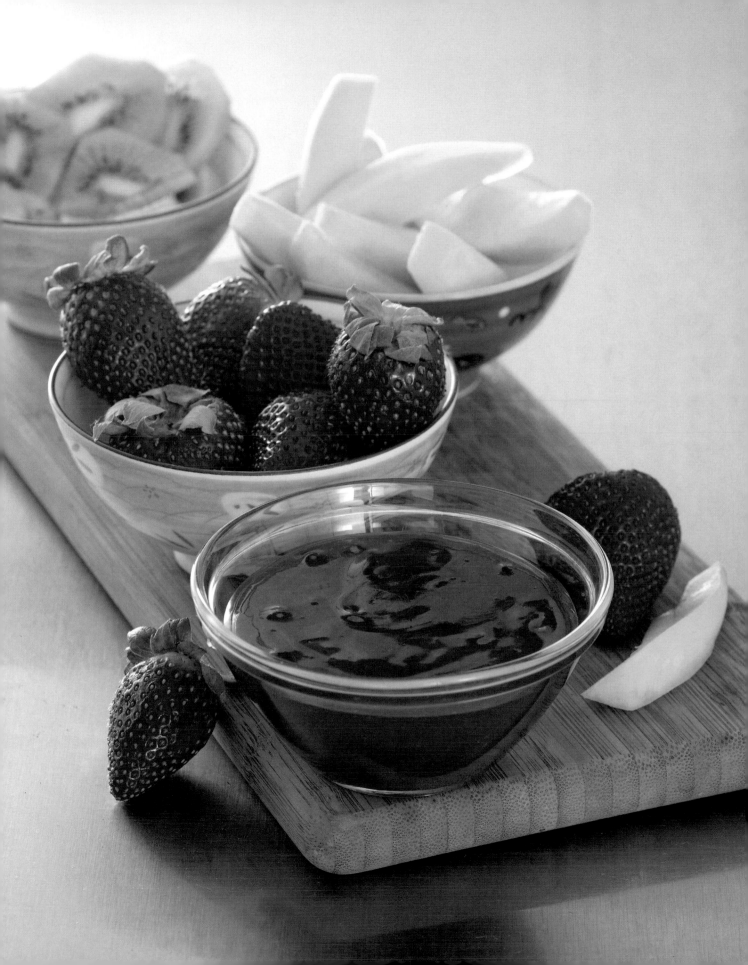

PART 2

PLAN MEALS
STRATEGICALLY

{ DAY 3 } Eat All Your Colors

NATURE PROVIDES A WIDE SPECTRUM of colorful fruits and vegetables, making it easy for you to get the variety of nutrients your body needs. Eating fruits and veggies of many colors is as important as eating five to nine servings each day. In our many years of working with schoolchildren of all ages, we've discovered we can get kids to eat new fruits and veggies by enticing them with colors.

eat with your eyes to get more nutrients

Just as insects are attracted to colorful flowers, we, too, "eat with our eyes." Research has shown that we respond positively to colorful stimuli. This is especially true of young children. If our food is visually appealing, we are more likely to eat it. By using color to make your family meals beautiful, you can shift your role from nutrition police officer to celebrated chef.

In our programs, "eating all your colors" is always the first lesson. Children are amazed and amused to discover purple carrots, rainbow chards, or yellow, orange, and green tomatoes. These surprising colors take away the threat of veggies.

We also encourage children to explore the produce with their hands, their lips, and *oops*, down the throat! But kids don't have to eat the veggies if they are not ready. Familiarity and a pleasurable experience are all they need at first.

eat a rainbow of colors to get the nutrients you need

The contemporary version of the old adage "eat an apple a day" is "eat a rainbow a day." Fruits and veggies are naturally low in fat. They provide a wide range of vitamins and minerals, as well as antioxidants and fiber. They boost your immune system and protect against aging, cancer, and heart disease. Scientific research has revealed that supplements do not provide the same benefits as eating the fresh fruits and veggies themselves. Why? Phytochemicals may be one of the answers.

Phytochemicals are microsubstances associated with health-promoting benefits found *only* in plant foods. Plants naturally produce these substances to protect themselves against viruses, bacteria, and fungi. Different plant foods contain different phytochemicals, depending on their color and plant family. Varying the colors you eat will ensure you get a wide range of phytochemicals, as well as other essential nutrients. This also helps protect your family from many diseases, including urinary tract problems, memory dysfunction, vision problems, and many cancers.

"eat all your colors" family challenge
try to serve an item from every color every day.

color	sun	mon	tues	wed	thurs	fri	sat
blue/purple blackberries, blueberries, eggplant, figs, grapes, plums, prunes, purple asparagus, purple cabbage, purple carrots, purple chard, purple potatoes, raisins							
green artichoke, arugula, asparagus, avocado, broccoli, broccoli rabe, brussels sprouts, celery, chard, collards, cucumber, endive, grapes, green apples, green beans, green pears, green peppers, greens, kale, kiwi, limes, peas, spinach, watercress							
white/brown bananas, brown pears, cauliflower, dates, garlic, ginger, leeks, mushrooms, onions, parsnips, potatoes, shallots, turnips, white nectarines, white peaches							
yellow/orange apricots, carrots, grapefruit, lemons, mangos, nectarines, oranges, papaya, peaches, persimmons, pineapples, pumpkins, spaghetti squash, squash, sweet potatoes/yams, tangerines							
red apples, beets, cherries, cranberries, pomegranates, radishes, raspberries, red cabbage, red onions, red peppers, rhubarb, strawberries, tomatoes, watermelon							

play color games to get kids to eat more vegetables

Rather than insisting kids eat veggies for health reasons, play games that encourage them to eat new fruits and vegetables. Here are some suggestions:

- ♡ Encourage children to explore the shapes and textures of exotic, colorful fruits and veggies. Slice and artfully arrange them on a tray.
- ♡ Do a fruit and vegetable tasting, by colors. Ask kids which color tastes more acidic (citrus), sweet (most ripe fruits), or bitter (arugula).
- ♡ Count the many colors in a mixed salad.
- ♡ Combine colors. Squeeze lemon (yellow) over a fruit medley (blueberries and red raspberries) and use as a topping for yogurt, pancakes, or oatmeal. For more color, add kiwi and banana.

The most successful strategy game in our program encourages eating "all your colors." The chart at left breaks down fruits and vegetables into color groups so you can keep track and shop for all colors. Photocopy this chart and hang it on your fridge.

When you shop, make it a game for your kids to choose items from every color column. Then use the chart to track what each person eats each day. If they eat a fruit or veggie from a color group on a particular day, put their initials in the box for that day. Portion size does not matter: if they taste one green pea, put their initials in the Green row.

Award two prizes: one to the person who eats the most produce and one to the person who eats the most colors. You'll be surprised at how eager children are to "eat all their colors" and beat Mom and Dad.

Hint: Keep fresh or frozen berries and a variety of dried fruits on hand so you have all the colors kids need to eat to "win" each day.

🕐 get started

Every recipe in this book offers a delicious opportunity to incorporate colorful fruits and vegetables into your diet. These can be varied by season, so you really have hundreds of recipes at your fingertips.

- ♡ Serve two veggies of different colors with your meals, on a plate whose color enhances the veggies.
- ♡ Start with foods your family likes and make them more fun and celebratory. For example, make your own tricolored baked french fries: purple (potatoes, when available), orange (yams), and white (potatoes).
- ♡ Surprise your family with orange mashed sweet potatoes.
- ♡ Arrange a plate of crudités of different colors and serve when kids are watching TV or playing with friends.
- ♡ Place bowls of colorful fruit conveniently around the house. You never know.

If you can achieve this step, you are halfway down the path to eating healthy for life.

fricassee of assorted seasonal greens and vegetables

Rainbow chard lets you get all your colors at once. The other veggies can be changed based on the season—be creative.

4 cups (896 g) rainbow chard or mixed greens (arugula, bok choy, mustard, mizuna, spinach, watercress, or collard), washed

1 cup (235 ml) chicken or vegetable broth

¼ cup (60 ml) extra-virgin olive oil

1 cup (70 g) mushrooms

1 medium zucchini

1 or 2 small orange and yellow bell peppers

½ cup (75 g) red and yellow cherry tomatoes

5 sprigs fresh basil or dill

Sautéed chicken thighs or legs, shrimp, scallops, or shellfish to add at the end of cooking for a full meal (optional)

NOTE: *Children should use plastic or table knives for all child steps that require cutting or chopping.*

CHILD Help tear the chard or other greens. Snap off the fibrous stems and discard.

ADULT Add the broth, olive oil, and greens to a large skillet over medium heat. Simmer for 3 minutes.

ADULT & CHILD Meanwhile, slice the mushrooms, gill side up; add mushrooms to the skillet and mix well. Cook for 2 minutes.

ADULT Slice the zucchini and bell peppers.

CHILD Dice the zucchini and bell peppers. Add to the skillet.

ADULT Mix well and cook for 3 minutes more. Remove from heat.

CHILD Help slice cherry tomatoes in half.

CHILD Remove basil or dill leaves from stems; chop herbs coarsely.

ADULT & CHILD Sprinkle herbs and tomatoes as a garnish over vegetable mixture and serve.

PREP TIME	COOK TIME	YIELD
20 to 30 minutes	10 minutes	4 to 6 servings

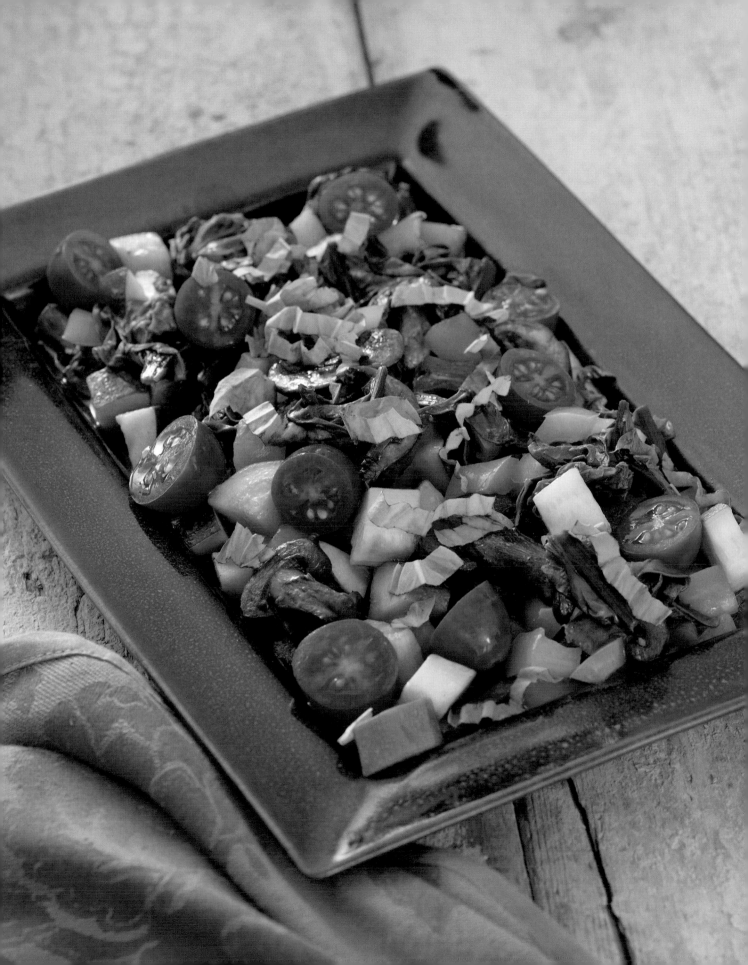

{ DAY 4 } Plan Meals Around Seasonal Foods

FOR MANY FAMILIES, meal planning is a dreaded task. Do you have children who will only eat a few dishes without a fuss? Lynn's two sons, when they were young, fit that description. Let's get real: As parents, we want to pick our battles, and mealtime isn't one of them. We believe the best way to approach the process of planning meals is to let the seasons be your guide. When you choose food according to the earth's cycles, your family's diet will naturally be well rounded.

fresh, seasonal produce is more interesting and tasty

Most supermarket fare appears seasonless—cherries in December, asparagus in January, and acorn squash

MISSION FOR THE DAY

Choose a vegetable that's only in season for a short time and use it to build your menu for dinner.

in May. You probably won't find much to inspire you there either because supermarkets and growers tend to select varieties that are hardy, rather than striving for diversity.

Fifteen years ago Lynn joined a Community Supported Agricultural (CSA) arrangement. This meant that in the spring she purchased a share in a regional farm's harvest. From June through November, she got weekly "harvest shares." Her first few shares contained veggies she had never heard of—sorrel and lamb's-quarters—but she learned how to prepare them. Her new recipes honored the seasonal fare. She also found she could reduce the cooking time for most summer veggies because they were so fresh and tender. She became a master at creating interesting salads and soups. The best new recipes became favorites that she adjusted as the seasons—and produce—changed.

Slowly, her children were won over because everything tasted so amazing! They learned that cherry tomatoes and snap peas were yummy for snacks. A big treat was a just-picked ear of sweet

grow a windowsill herb garden

Fresh herbs make a huge difference in recipes. Here's a way to ensure you have fresh seasonal herbs readily available: Store fresh herbs in glass jars or vases, like flowers. If you place them in a sunny window and change the water frequently, they often root. Pluck off tasty leaves of thyme, basil, or cilantro and add them to recipes; let children snip the leaves with kitchen shears.

ten ways to eat seasonally

1 As a family, look through our recipe concepts in the next chapter or your own recipes.

2 Choose seasonally appropriate recipes and variations for three days.

3 Give preference to recipes that use produce that is only in season for a short time.

4 Use vegetables from your community-supported agriculture (CSA) share in the recipe.

5 Plan a trip to the farmers' market to experience the types and variety of locally grown seasonal produce, or look for signs at your supermarket that indicate local produce.

6 Use the "Eat All Your Colors" chart in Day 3 when you shop, to get items from each color category.

7 Don't wait until you are starving or tired after a day at work to start preparing vegetables. Trim, cut, and chop vegetables to use later in the week. Invite your kids to assist you. Wrap the veggies in a damp paper towel and place in a plastic bag or in a humidity-controlled section of your fridge.

8 When you try something new and your family loves it, take a photo, or have a youngster draw the food, then post the picture on your fridge.

9 The weekly food section of your local newspaper offers great seasonal recipes. Start a family challenge. Let a different member of the family choose a recipe each week to make.

10 When you go to the source, you get the best information. If there is a vegetable you love but don't know how to prepare it, or one you cook all the time and need some new ideas for using it, ask the farmers at the farmers' market. They are a treasure trove of ideas, information, and recipes.

corn. When a farmers' market opened a few blocks away from her home, Lynn knew to look out for pea shoots and ramps in May as the first signs that the earth was waking up after the long winter's sleep. One fall Lynn's son Stephan volunteered to meet her at the market and carry the heavy bag of apples home on the handlebars of his bike. His incentive? Her delicious apple pie.

Seasons came to mean something to her boys: The first strawberries, cherries, snap peas, and peaches were something to celebrate. Fresh seasonal herbs perfumed her kitchen. Food shopping became exciting because every week something new appeared.

Eating seasonally has been a hallmark of our educational programs for children of all ages. This lets children enjoy different tastes and associate various recipes and flavors with the time of year. We don't make butternut squash soup in May, and we don't make tomato salad in December.

Before food became artificially available at any time of year, nature wisely designed our food supply to provide us with a healthy diet. Until recently, people around the world ate seasonally, and doing so balanced their diets and their bodies. Eating by the seasons may sound limiting and unrealistic, but trust us, it's the most wonderful way to enjoy a varied diet. It also lets you easily replicate your meal-planning strategy year after year.

In different regions, fruits and vegetables grow at different times of the year. Watch your local farmers' market to see what's available when, and design colorful meals accordingly. As you become familiar with what grows when, you'll find exciting

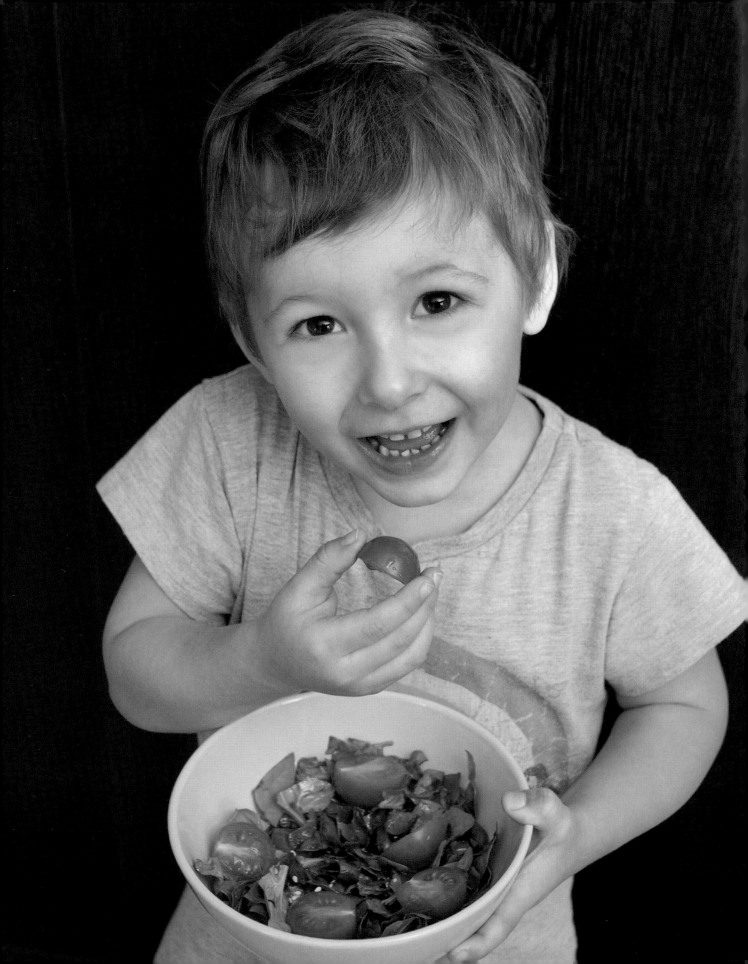

ways to shop for seasonal produce and make great-tasting meals that combine festive colors. To find out what's in season in your area, contact your local agricultural department. You can also download the Seasons app (www.seasonsapp.com) if you have an iPhone.

entice your children to snack on fresh fruits and veggies

"Advertise" to your family that you've shopped at the farmers' market. By keeping bowls of fresh produce around your home, you signal that these fruits and vegetables are there to be eaten. By surrounding kids with tempting, seasonal, and healthy food, they never have to open a fridge or a cabinet if they are hungry.

get started

Luckily, the public health community is focusing on providing better access to seasonal fresh food. Now it's easier to find stores and markets that prioritize what's in season. Here are some ways to locate and use seasonal fresh produce:

- Give priority to recipes that use vegetables available only briefly.
- Visit www.localharvest.org to find the best options for local produce in your area.
- Visit the website of your state agricultural department for information about what grows when in your region.
- Plan a trip to the farmers' market to experience the varieties and types of produce grown locally. Taste farm fresh veggies raw; dip veggies into hummus or salsa.

Watch your local farmers' market to see what's available when, and design colorful meals accordingly.

summer flan with heirloom tomatoes

In this recipe you can taste summer on a plate. Sweet, fresh zucchini transforms into a delightful flan. Use any ripe heirloom tomato variety for this recipe.

2 to 3 pounds (910 g to 1.4 kg) zucchini

1½ tablespoons (27 g) sea salt

½ teaspoon herbs de Provence

½ cup (120 ml) extra-virgin olive oil, divided

2 large cloves garlic

½ tablespoon butter

5 eggs

¼ cup (60 ml) cream or milk

2 large ripe heirloom tomatoes

5 sprigs fresh basil

½ tablespoon agave syrup or sugar, or to taste

ADDITIONAL COOKING EQUIPMENT:
9 x 5 x 3-inch (23 x 13 x 7.5 cm) loaf pan; larger baking dish loaf pan will fit into

NOTE: *Children should use plastic or table knives for all child steps that require cutting or chopping.*

ADULT Preheat oven to 350°F (180°C, or gas mark 4). Wash all the vegetables. Cut the zucchini into thirds. Cut each third in half lengthwise. Thinly slice each zucchini section, flat side down.

CHILD Measure the salt and herbs de Provence and combine in a small mixing bowl. Sprinkle zucchini slices with the seasoned salt. Set aside.

ADULT Heat ¼ cup (60 ml) of the olive oil in a large skillet over medium heat. Add the seasoned zucchini slices to the pan sauté.

ADULT & CHILD Adult smashes the garlic with the flat side of a chef's knife to remove the peel. Adult slices and child helps chop it finely.

ADULT Add the garlic to the zucchini and stir to incorporate well. Adjust heat so zucchini slices become limp but do not change color.

ADULT & CHILD Child lightly greases the loaf pan with the butter. Adult uses a flexible spatula to transfer the zucchini to a paper towel to absorb excess moisture.

ADULT & CHILD In a mixing bowl, combine eggs and cream. Mix well. Carefully add cooked zucchini slices to the egg mixture.

ADULT Pour mixture into the prepared loaf pan. Place the loaf pan into a large baking dish with 3-inch (7.5 cm) sides. Boil water and pour it into the larger baking dish until it reaches up to half the height of the loaf pan. (This prevents custard from forming a crust.) Bake in the preheated oven for about 30 minutes, or until set.

ADULT & CHILD While the flan is baking, adult slices tomatoes and child cuts them into cubes by stacking the slices.

ADULT In a small skillet, add the tomatoes and the remaining olive oil.

CHILD Remove basil leaves from stems and tear up leaves. Add to tomatoes. Measure agave and add.

ADULT Cook and stir the tomatoes over medium heat until they break down and form a sauce. Add more seasoned salt to taste.

ADULT Unmold the flan onto a rectangular or oval serving platter. Pour the tomato sauce over it. Slice and serve with a spoonful of sauce over each serving.

PREP TIME	COOK TIME	YIELD
20 minutes	30 minutes	4 to 6 servings

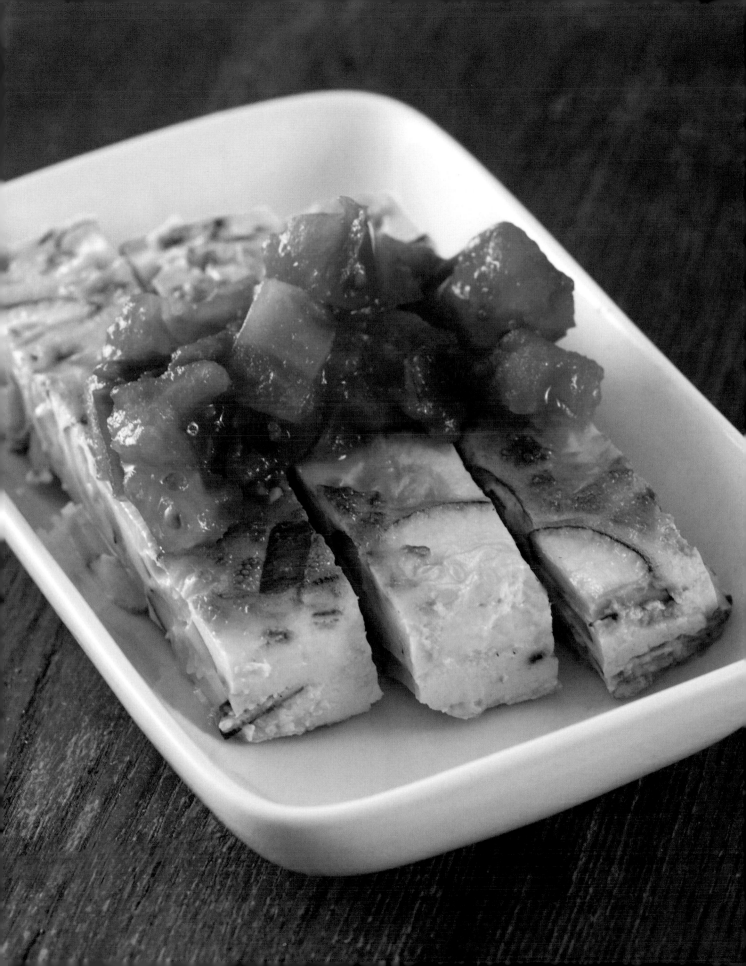

festive roasted fall vegetables

For the most appealing result, select root veggies of contrasting colors. You can leave the peels on all the veggies—even the acorn squash. Just scrub them well, and make sure you cut the squash into semicircles for easy prep and beauty on the plate.

1 medium potato

1 medium sweet potato

4 small shallots

1 medium acorn or delicata squash

2 small parsnips

2 small turnips

¼ cup (60 ml) olive oil

Salt and freshly ground black pepper

6 tablespoons (85 g) unsalted butter

3 to 4 fresh sage leaves

1 to 2 teaspoons Spanish sherry vinegar

ADDITIONAL COOKING EQUIPMENT:
Baking sheet or roasting pan

NOTE: *Children should use plastic or table knives for all child steps that require cutting or chopping.*

ADULT Preheat oven to 400 °F (200°C, or gas mark 6)

ADULT & CHILD Adult slices the vegetables. Child can then cut into bite-size and attractive-looking pieces.

ADULT & CHILD Place the vegetables in a large bowl, add olive oil, and season to taste with salt and pepper. Toss.

ADULT Spread the vegetables on an oiled baking sheet. Bake in the preheated oven for 30 minutes, or until vegetables are caramelized (browned or roasted to sweetness).

ADULT Meanwhile, melt the butter in a small skillet over medium heat.

CHILD Tear up sage leaves and add to the skillet.

ADULT Cook until the butter browns but does not burn. Remove from heat; add the vinegar and season with salt to taste.

ADULT Serve by placing each portion of veggies on its own plate. Drizzle just enough of the sherry-sage butter over the veggies to add taste—don't drench.

PREP TIME	COOK TIME	YIELD
20 minutes	30 minutes	4 to 6 servings

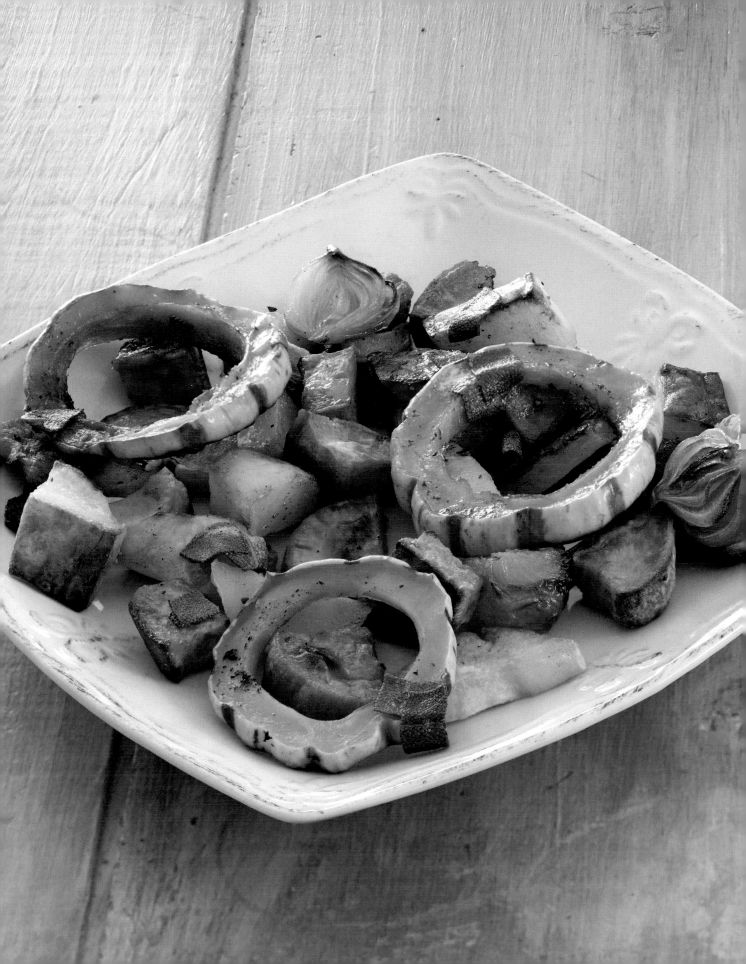

winter squash bread pudding

Bread pudding is a delectable and inexpensive dessert. This version adds nutrition and sneaks in those veggies. It's a nice alternative to banana or zucchini bread.

1 large acorn squash or small butternut squash

1 baguette, day old and hard, or toasted in oven

1 cup (235 ml) heavy cream

½ cup (120 ml) milk, whole or 2 percent fat

½ cup (100 g) sugar

1 teaspoon ground cinnamon

½ teaspoon ground ginger

⅛ teaspoon ground nutmeg

⅛ teaspoon ground cloves

⅛ teaspoon ground allspice

3 large eggs

1 egg yolk

4 tablespoons (55 g) butter

Fresh cream for garnish (optional)

ADDITIONAL COOKING EQUIPMENT:
10 x 8 x 2-inch (25 x 20 x 5 cm) baking dish (slightly larger is fine)

NOTE: *Children should use plastic or table knives for all child steps that require cutting or chopping.*

ADULT Preheat oven to 350 °F (180°C, or gas mark 4).

ADULT Cut the squash in half and remove seeds. Place both halves cut side down in a 10 x 8 x 2-inch (25 x 20 x 5 cm) baking dish; add ½ inch (13 mm) of water. Roast in preheated oven about 40 minutes, or until tender.

ADULT & CHILD While the squash is roasting, adult slices the bread, and child cuts the slices into 1-inch (2.5 cm) cubes until there are 6 cups (355 g) of cubed bread.

ADULT & CHILD Measure the cream, milk, sugar, cinnamon, ginger, nutmeg, cloves, and allspice and place in a large mixing bowl. Add the eggs and egg yolk and whisk thoroughly.

ADULT Melt the butter in a medium saucepan. Add the bread cubes and toss until coated.

ADULT Remove squash from the oven. Cool.

CHILD Scoop out the roasted squash from the shell. Add to the bread mixture in the saucepan. Mix well. Add the egg mixture and mix well.

ADULT Pour mixture into the same ungreased baking dish. Bake in the preheated oven 25 to 30 minutes, or until the custard is set.

ADULT Serve warm with a drizzle of fresh cream.

PREP TIME	COOK TIME	YIELD
10 minutes	40 minutes to roast squash (can be done in advance); 25 to 30 minutes to cook the pudding	8 servings

{DAY 5} Choose Recipes by Concept

PLANNING MEALS day after day is a chore most of us find daunting and tedious. The secret to making the meal-planning process more fun and exciting involves learning recipes concepts that can be adapted to what's in season as well as your family's preferences. These concepts are one-pot or one-bowl dishes that hail from around the globe. Quiche, stew, risotto, fricassee, quesadilla, and composed salads—we offer lots of different options that your family can experiment with. Vary these dishes depending on the season, and make them your own.

We have tested these concepts in our FamilyCook programs for many years, and they appeal to all ages. Children love them because there are lots of ingredients they can explore and experience. Parents love their flexibility because they can leave out the green beans from a composed salad, for instance, and substitute broccoli or a family favorite

MISSION
FOR THE DAY

For dinner, adapt a concept to the current season.

that's in season. Selecting menus by concept eliminates the stress and limitation of designing menus for picky eaters.

Planning meals with recipe concepts offers many other benefits, too:

- ♡ The concepts use minimal meat, so you save money.
- ♡ Our colorful dishes celebrate various cultures.
- ♡ You can create infinite variations once you get the hang of each concept. Mealtime need never be dull again.
- ♡ Most, but not quite all our concepts, can be made quickly and require only basic cooking tools and a few appliances.
- ♡ Most of our concepts include food from all the food groups, or you can easily add a grain or some plant-based or animal protein to make a balanced meal.
- ♡ Because each recipe uses multiple seasonal vegetables, there are lots of fun tasks for kids, such as chopping, grating, measuring, and peeling.

To make it easy for families to follow these steps, we've introduced a range of delicious, kid-friendly, crowd-pleasing recipe concepts—all with seasonal variations. In our eighteen years of using

how to plan seasonal family meals

- Choose a seasonal vegetable for your family to try.

- Decide what recipes you make or want to try that can use these seasonal vegetables. (Use the chart in this chapter to get started.)

- Plan three days' worth of meals you can make by varying the protein and grains around these seasonal foods.

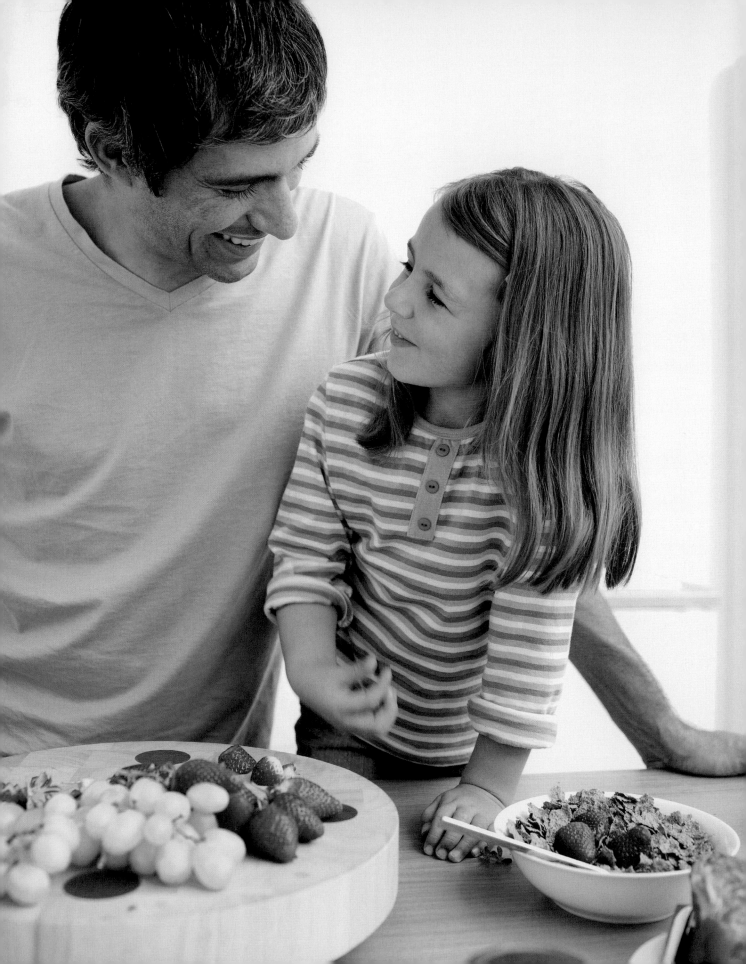

example: recipe concepts with seasonal variations

fruits and their concepts	spring	summer	fall	winter
muffins (day 7) pancakes (day 25) smoothie (day 27)	Rhubarb, strawberries	Apricots, blueberries, cherries, currents, grapes, nectarines, peaches, plums, raspberries	Apples, cranberries, grapes, figs, homemade applesauce, pears	Bananas, dates, frozen berries, nuts, tropical fruits

vegetables and their concepts	spring	summer	fall	winter
bread salad (day 15) omelet (day 25) quesadilla (day 5) pasta (day 23) pureed soups (day 14) quiche (day 9) risotto (day 20) wrap sandwiches (day 28)	Asparagus, cranberry and fava beans, cucumbers, garlic scapes, greens, herbs, morel mushrooms, peas and pea shoots, ramps	Basil, bell peppers, broccoli, cauliflower, chili peppers, corn, cucumbers, greens (chards, collards, kale, mustard, spinach), herbs, leeks, snap peas, string beans, summer squash, tomatoes	Brussels sprouts, herbs, kales, leeks, mushrooms, potatoes, root vegetables, tomatoes, winter squash (acorn, butternut, delicata)	Canned tomatoes, dried mushrooms, leeks, potatoes, root vegetables, winter kale and squashes

these recipe concepts, families in our programs have thanked us for freeing them from being slaves to recipes. With a little advanced planning, you will rely on quick packaged solutions less often and try new recipes more frequently.

In the chart above, we have listed some examples of recipe concepts that you'll find in this book, as well as the chapters where they appear. Not all of the recipes are listed here; however, there are just enough to give you a good idea of how to start. You can adjust the seasonal ingredients and vary the plant or animal protein for diversity.

get started

When you first start to use the strategy of recipe concepts, this chart can be helpful. Here are some other tips to help you plan your meals:

♡ Browse the concepts in the book and select one.
♡ Consider the staples you have on hand.
♡ Choose what's most appealing from the current season's fresh produce in our chart.
♡ Make a trip to a farmers' market if necessary for the freshest seasonal ingredients.

The following recipes will give you an understanding of how to work with a basic concept and vary it for different meals, seasons, and your family's preferences. The recipe concept example used here is the quesadilla, which hails from Mexico. You can keep quesadillas in the fridge or freezer; they make great quick meals and snacks, combined with leftover meat or veggies and flavorings such as hummus, guacamole, mashed canned beans, roasted peppers, olives, or tomatoes.

fig and goat cheese quesadilla

This unique recipe gives the typical quesadilla a Middle Eastern twist. It's delicious for breakfast any time of the year. You can substitute other seasonal fruit or jam, such as plums, raspberries, or peaches.

4 whole wheat tortillas

Fig jam

4 ounces (115 g) goat cheese

NOTE: *Children should use plastic or table knives for all child steps that require cutting or chopping.*

CHILD Place 2 tortillas on a clean table or cutting board.

CHILD Spread fig jam over the tortillas in a thin, even layer.

ADULT & CHILD Distribute chunks of goat cheese evenly over the fruit. Place the remaining 2 tortillas on top and press down firmly.

ADULT Heat a dry cast-iron skillet over high heat, and cook the quesadillas, one at a time, until browned on the bottom. Then carefully flip it over with a spatula so the second side can brown. (If it starts to burn, the temperature is too high.)

ADULT Use a spatula to transfer each cooked quesadilla to a plate and cover with foil to keep warm.

PREP TIME	COOK TIME	YIELD
5 minutes	5 minutes	4 servings of ½ quesadilla each

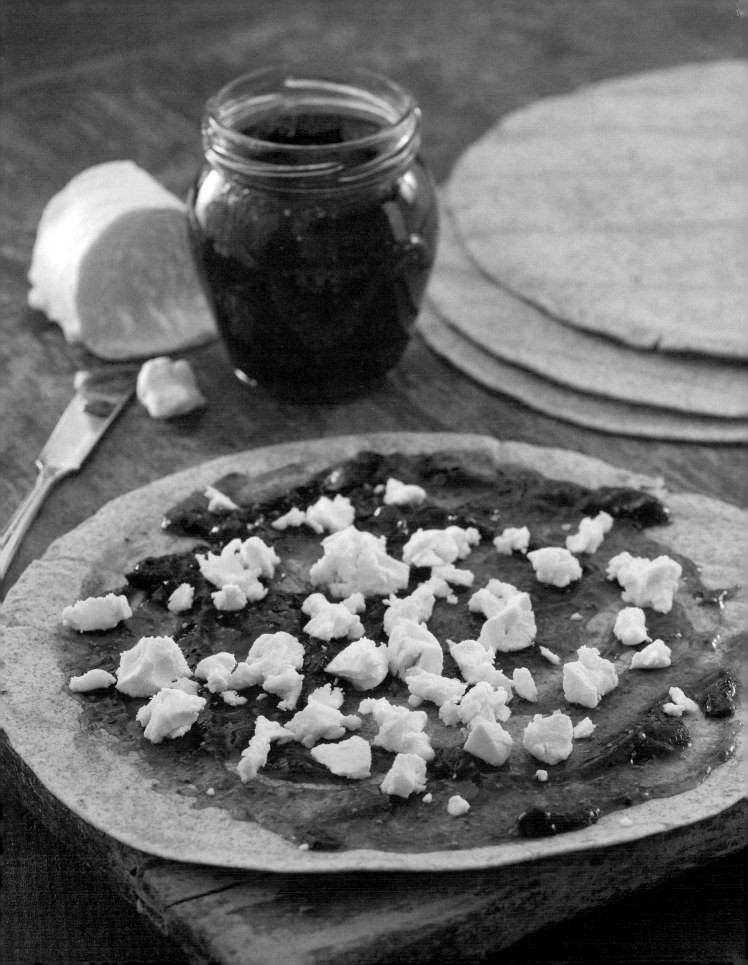

veggie quesadillas

Quesadillas are a great strategy to use up leftovers. You can put just about any leftover meat or veggie in this recipe to develop your own original creations. You can also add mashed beans for a nutritious combination.

8 flour tortillas, 8 or 10 inches (20 or 25 cm) in diameter

8 ounces (225 g) cheese #1 (Monterey Jack, cheddar, asadero)

8 ounces (225 g) cheese #2 (any other cheese you like)

½ bunch seasonal greens (mustard, chard, kale) or a mixture

1 jar (4 ounces, or 115 g) pesto, almond butter, hummus, or salsa, or 3 mashed avocados

⅓ cup (50 g) seasonal vegetables (asparagus, beets, turnips, carrots) or a mixture

Slices of cooked chicken, turkey, ham, or sausage, or smoked salmon (optional)

Sour cream, cilantro leaves, or fresh guacamole for garnish

ADDITIONAL COOKING EQUIPMENT:
10-inch (25 -cm) cast iron skillet or cooking spray for regular skillet

NOTE: *Children should use plastic or table knives for all child steps that require cutting or chopping.*

CHILD Place 4 flour tortillas on a clean table or cutting board.

ADULT & CHILD Grate or crumble cheese #1 into a bowl.

ADULT & CHILD Grate or crumble cheese #2 into a separate bowl.

ADULT Steam the greens. Remove and cool for 5 to 10 minutes. Squeeze out excess liquid and chop.

CHILD Spread a generous layer of the pesto, almond butter, hummus, salsa, or mashed avocados over each tortilla. Then sprinkle some chopped greens on top.

ADULT & CHILD Grate or chop the veggies and sprinkle over the chopped greens on the quesadilla.

ADULT & CHILD Sprinkle ½ cup (56 g) of grated or crumbled cheese #1 evenly over each tortilla, followed by ½ cup (56 g) of cheese #2.

CHILD Place another flour tortilla over each quesadilla and press it down firmly over the filling.

ADULT Heat a large dry cast iron skillet over medium-high heat and cook the quesadillas, one at a time, until browned on the bottom. Then carefully flip it over with a spatula so the second side can brown. (If it starts to burn, the temperature is too high.)

ADULT Use a spatula to transfer each quesadilla to a plate and cover with foil to keep warm. Repeat until all the quesadillas are cooked.

ADULT Cut into wedges and serve warm with desired garnish.

PREP TIME	COOK TIME	YIELD
15 minutes	10 minutes	8 servings of ½ quesadilla each

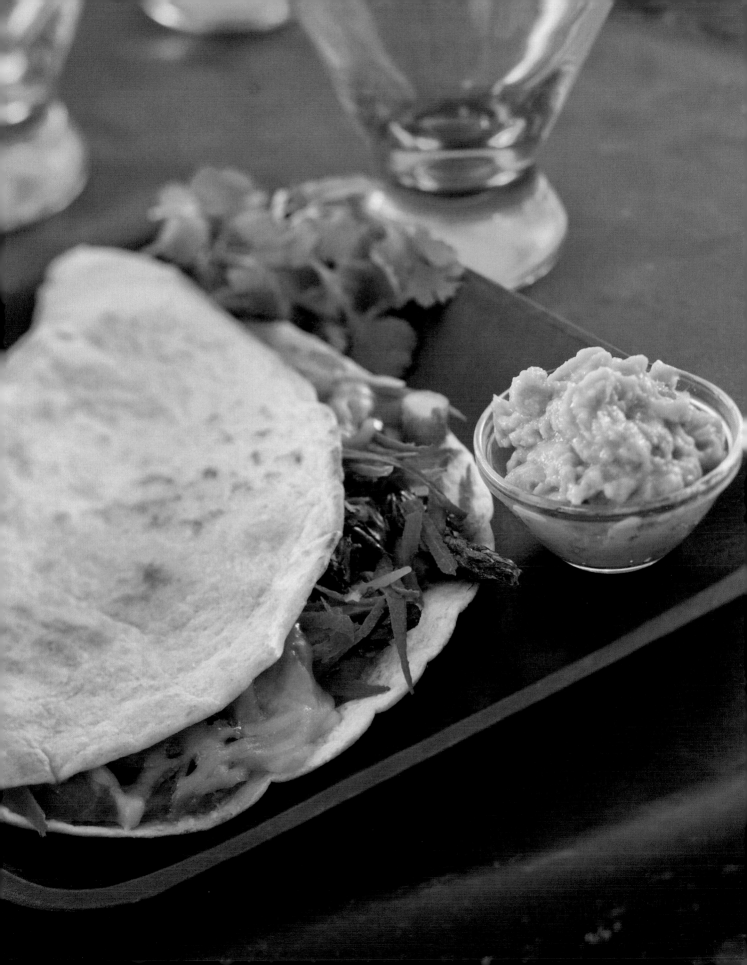

rainbow chard and apple quesadillas

This is an unusual way to eat delicious Swiss chard. The sweetness of the apples and cider make it irresistible to all ages.

1 bunch rainbow chard

1 medium onion

3 tablespoons (45 ml) olive oil

3 apples

⅓ cup (80 ml) apple cider

Salt and pepper

8 flour tortillas, 8 or 10 inches (20 to 25 cm) in diameter

8 ounces (225 g) goat cheese

NOTE: *Children should use plastic or table knives for all child steps that require cutting or chopping.*

CHILD Snap the stems from the chard and discard.

ADULT Slice onion into pieces children can cut. Neatly stack the chard leaves, 3 or 4 at a time, and slice into ½-inch (13 mm) ribbons. Continue until all the chard is sliced.

ADULT & CHILD Dice the onion very fine.

ADULT Heat the olive oil in a medium saucepan over high heat. Add the onions, reduce heat to low, and cook, stirring frequently, about 10 minutes, or until onions are translucent.

ADULT & CHILD Meanwhile, peel, core, and dice the apples.

ADULT Add the apples and cider to the saucepan. Cook 5 minutes, or until apples are tender. Remove from heat.

ADULT Measure 10 ounces (280 ml) water into a medium saucepan and bring to boil. Place rainbow chard in the boiling water and blanch for 90 seconds. Remove the chard with tongs and cool in a bowl of ice water. Reserve the cooking water.

CHILD Remove chard from bowl and place on paper towels. Gently help squeeze the excess water from the chard.

CHILD Add the chard to the apple mixture and mix well.

ADULT Add ⅓ cup (80 ml) of the cooking water to the apple mixture. Mix thoroughly. Season to taste with salt and pepper.

CHILD Place 4 tortillas on a clean table or cutting board. Divide the goat cheese into 4 equal portions, and spread one portion over each of the 4 tortillas.

ADULT & CHILD Evenly distribute the chard and apple mixture over each quesadilla. Place another flour tortilla over each quesadilla and press it down firmly over the filling.

Refer to page 42 for cooking instructions.

PREP TIME	COOK TIME	YIELD
15 minutes	20 minutes	4 quesadillas, or 8 to 16 servings depending on accompaniments

{ DAY 6 } Practice Savvy Seasonal Shopping and Save Money

WHEN YOU SHIFT YOUR FOCUS to eating whole, seasonal, local, and unprocessed foods, you'll approach shopping a bit differently. Your goal is to purchase the healthiest ingredients at an affordable price, which means you will rely *less* on one-stop supermarket shopping—at least part of the year—than you've done in the past.

buy higher quality food to support better health

American families spend a lower percentage of their incomes on food than do people in many other parts of the world. That's because we have lots of inexpensive food options—but they aren't necessarily the healthiest options. Of course, everyone has a budget, and it's a big factor in how you shop. That's why we offer recipes that are delicious and satisfying, as well as economical. We suggest you buy high-quality produce and dairy products, but you'll compensate for the extra cost by replacing some of the expensive animal protein you've been eating with inexpensive legumes and grains. Consider it an investment.

> **MISSION FOR THE DAY**
>
> Find a store nearby that offers a good selection of locally grown and unprocessed foods.

We both raised children in New York City, where quality food can be pretty costly. Hence, we frequent a variety of stores so we get quality whole foods for the best price. Because we prioritize what to buy seasonally, we shop at the farmers' market for most seasonal vegetables, dairy products, and some seafood and meats. About once a month, we stock up on staples, produce, organic meat, and frozen line-caught fish from health-focused retailers that offer good value. There we also buy quality prepared foods, such as dumplings and tamales made with whole, natural ingredients, for those times when we need to make quick meals. We supplement with food from the local supermarket and specialty stores, taking into consideration money-saving promotions and specific ingredients needed for the recipes we plan to prepare.

stock up on staples to save time and money

When we did some comparison shopping, we found we often saved two to three dollars per staple item simply by shopping at several stores. Yes, we know, it seems like a lot of extra shopping time, but don't be intimidated; you can compare items in a single trip and make note of which store is best for staples, then purchase weekly or monthly. We suggest stocking up on these staples: dried fruits, nuts, legumes, oils, vinegars, spices, salt, sugar, flour, nut butters, dry and canned tomatoes (whole and crushed), vegetable and chicken stock, whole grains (quinoa, one or more types of rice, barley), pasta and other noodles, jams, whole-grain cereals (minimally processed), tea, coffee, and frozen fruits, vegetables, fish, and meat.

When you shop, look for these items:

- ♡ locally grown produce, meat, and dairy products (organic or at least without hormones and antibiotics)
- ♡ organic foods
- ♡ whole and minimally processed foods
- ♡ foods with few or no additives
- ♡ seafood that is wild, not farmed, and line caught

Organic food—especially produce—is becoming cheaper. Supermarkets often have their own organic brands that offer the best value. In many supermarkets you'll find organic dairy products (milk, cheese, eggs, yogurt), fruit and vegetables, grains, canned goods, and meat, especially chicken.

We suggest you prioritize where you shop, and follow this order as much as possible:

1. Farmers' market or CSA
2. Health food stores
3. Supermarkets
4. Convenience stores

take a family field trip to the farmers' market

The farmers' market is the best resource for food education—and it's free! Everyone learns what's in season by taking in all the sights and smells. Often you'll find fresh foods to sample. If you have a question, just ask the farmer! Here are some topics you may want to discuss with your children:

- ♡ Explain that the earth's annual cycle is similar to our daily routine: We wake up in the morning and start the day anew; we are in full form midday; we wind down in the evening; and we sleep at night; and then we start the cycle again.
- ♡ Discuss foods that can and cannot grow in your climate.
- ♡ Explain that, in many parts of the world, during winter the earth is asleep and nothing grows. So at that time, we eat fresh foods such as root vegetables, apples, and squash that have "winter coats" and can be stored over the winter.
- ♡ In spring the earth wakes up, and new plants and foods appear, such as peas and rhubarb.
- ♡ In fall, after the final harvest is in, the earth begins to wind down and prepare for its winter rest.

We suggest you buy high-quality produce and dairy products, but you'll compensate for the extra cost by replacing some of the expensive animal protein you've been eating with inexpensive legumes and grains.

⏱ get started

Go at your own pace—you don't have to do everything at once:

- ♡ Select some staples you buy regularly and compare their prices between the store where you usually shop and one that's new to you.
- ♡ Ask at your farmers' market if locally produced meat or fish is available.
- ♡ Explore local resources for eggs and dairy products, comparing prices and convenience.
- ♡ Assess the options available to you for purchasing healthy, whole foods. Where you shop will likely change at different times of the year, based on seasonal availability, your schedule, and even the weather.

- ♡ Go online to www.farmersmarket.com or www.localharvest.org to locate a farmers' market or CSA near you.
- ♡ Check www.coopdirectory.org/directory.htm to find a food cooperative or buying club that can help you save money and get excellent quality.
- ♡ Go to health-focused supermarkets.
- ♡ Visit specialty stores near you.
- ♡ If possible, purchase organic, minimally processed, and additive-free foods at supermarket chains.

snap pea and mint pasta

This pasta dish includes a refreshing hint of mint. It's also a wonderful way to enjoy fresh snap peas in the spring.

SEASON: Spring

¾ pound (340 g) snap peas

½ tablespoon salt

½ pound (225 g) farfalle or bow tie pasta

½ bunch fresh mint

2 tablespoons (30 ml) olive oil

Salt and pepper

1 oz (28 g) Parmesan cheese, or other hard cheese, grated

ADDITIONAL COOKING EQUIPMENT:
Cheese grater

NOTE: *Children should use plastic or table knives for all child steps that require cutting or chopping.*

ADULT & CHILD Remove the strip of membrane on the side of the snap peas.

ADULT Bring 3 quarts (2.8 L) of water to boil over high heat in a large saucepan and add the ½ tablespoon salt. Add the peas and boil for 2 minutes. Use a sieve or slotted spoon to remove the peas, reserving the water, and plunge them into a bowl of ice water to stop the cooking process.

ADULT Bring the reserved water back to a boil. Add the pasta and cook about 8 minutes, or until just cooked through but not mushy.

ADULT & CHILD Meanwhile, separate the mint leaves from the stems. Chop the leaves. Place in a serving bowl.

ADULT Drain the snap peas and add to the serving bowl.

ADULT Drain the cooked pasta and add to the serving bowl.

ADULT & CHILD Measure the olive oil. Pour it over the veggies and pasta; mix well. Grate cheese over each bowl. Season to taste with salt and pepper. Serve as a main dish, with a salad or side dish.

PREP TIME	COOK TIME	YIELD
10 minutes	10 minutes	4 servings

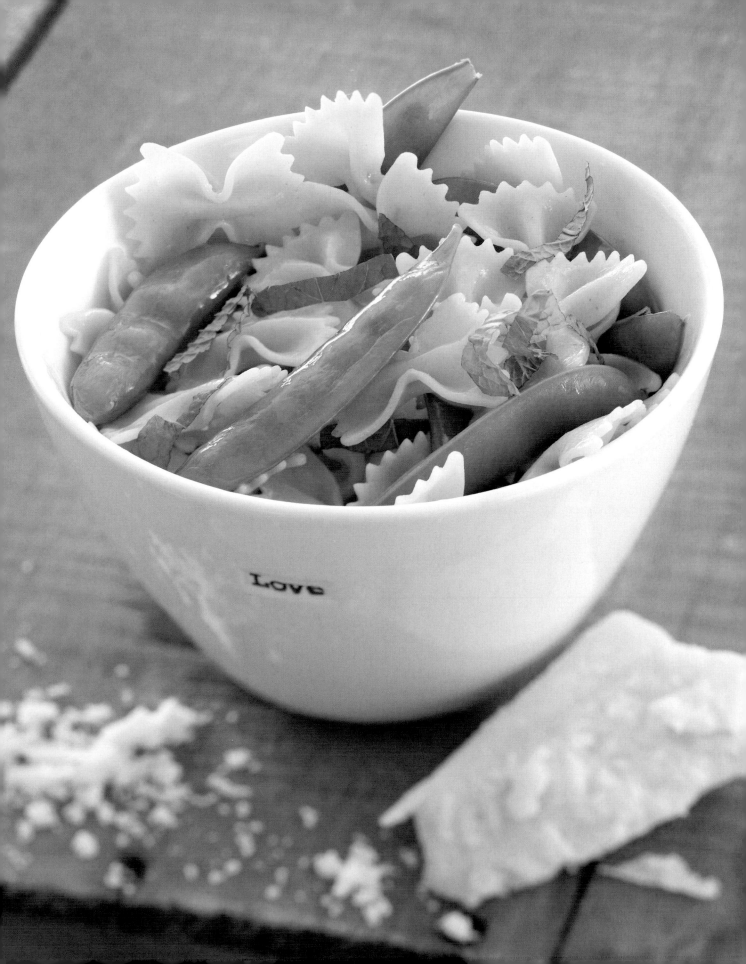

venezuelan arepas (corn pancakes)

This recipe is a crowd pleaser. It's best made with tender farm-fresh sweet corn in the summer. In the winter, use canned corn—it's a welcome reminder of warm, sunny days.

SEASON: Summer

2 ears sweet corn, shucked, or 1 can (15 ounces, or 420 g) corn

2 tablespoons (28 g) butter

⅓ cup (47 g) yellow cornmeal

½ cup (60 g) flour

1 teaspoon sugar

1 teaspoon salt

½ teaspoon baking soda

2 scallions

½ jalapeño pepper

½ red or orange bell pepper

1 large egg

½ cup (120 ml) milk

Peanut or canola oil, for cooking

½ cup (115 g) sour cream (optional)

4 tablespoons (4 g) cilantro, chopped (optional)

NOTE: *Children should use plastic or table knives for all child steps that require cutting or chopping.*

ADULT Slice the bottom of the corn off the cob and stand it up on the flat bottom. Slice the corn kernels off the cob and place into a large mixing bowl. Melt the butter in the microwave and set aside.

ADULT & CHILD Measure the cornmeal, flour, sugar, salt, and baking soda into the mixing bowl with the corn.

ADULT Slice the scallions and add to the corn mixture. Seed and mince the jalapeños (make sure you wear plastic gloves when preparing) and add to the corn mixture.

ADULT Slice the bell pepper into strips and then cut the slices into tiny pieces. Add to the corn mixture.

ADULT & CHILD In a separate bowl, whisk together the egg, milk, and melted butter.

ADULT & CHILD Pour the egg mixture into the corn mixture and mix well with a spoon.

ADULT Heat about 3 tablespoons (45 ml) oil in large skillet over medium-high heat. Spoon a heaping tablespoon of corn batter into the oil and spread the batter to form a pancake about 3½ inches (9 cm) across, using oven mitts to protect hands from heat.

ADULT Cook the pancake on one side until set, and then flip and continue cooking until lightly browned, 2 to 3 minutes on each side. Add additional oil if necessary. Drain pancakes on paper towels and keep warm. Continue until you have used all the batter.

ADULT & CHILD To serve, place 2 or 3 pancakes on each serving plate. If desired, spoon a little sour cream on the center or side of each pancake and top with some cilantro. Serve immediately as a side dish or in lieu of bread.

PREP TIME	COOK TIME	YIELD
15 minutes	15 minutes	6 servings of 2 pancakes each

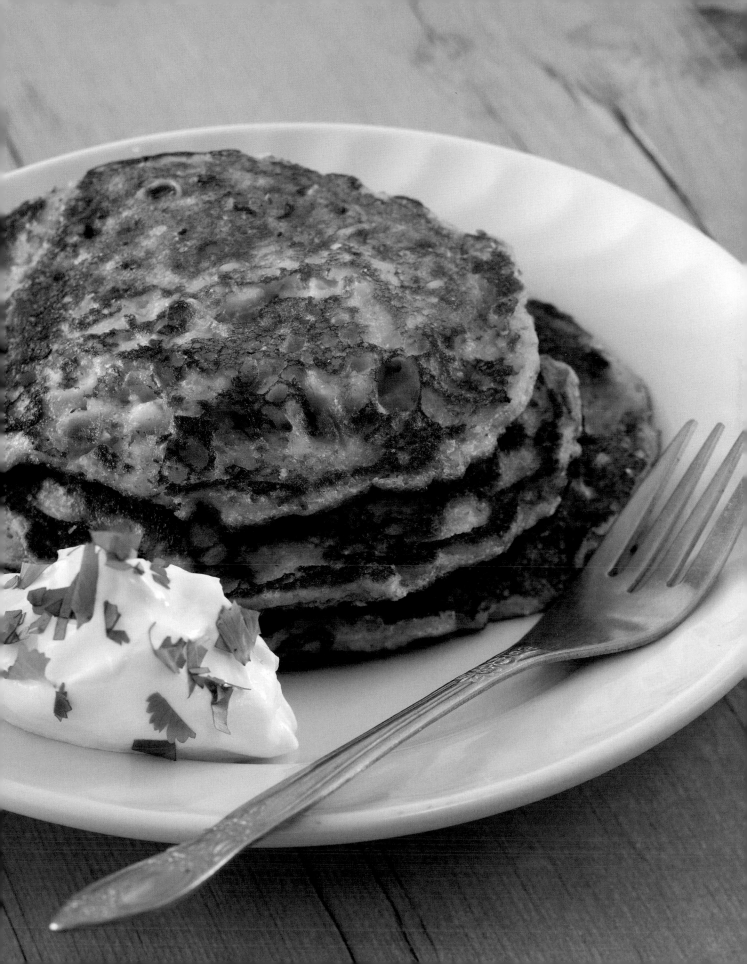

baked apples

Enjoy this tasty treat for dessert or as a snack.
SEASON: Fall or Winter

4 apples

1 tablespoon (15 ml) butter

¼ teaspoon ground cinnamon

2 tablespoons (18 g) raisins

2 tablespoons (30 g) packed brown sugar, or 1 tablespoon (15 ml) maple syrup

2 tablespoons (30 ml) crème fraîche or sour cream (optional)

ADDITIONAL COOKING EQUIPMENT: Baking pan large enough to fit the apples in.

NOTE: *Children should use plastic or table knives for all child steps that require cutting or chopping.*

ADULT Preheat oven to 350 °F (180°C, or gas mark 4). Core the apples and place in a baking dish.

CHILD Help measure the butter. Divide into 4 equal pieces. Push 1 piece of butter into the empty core of each apple.

ADULT & CHILD Measure the cinnamon. Distribute the cinnamon equally inside each of the 4 apples.

ADULT & CHILD Measure the raisins. Distribute the raisins equally inside each of the 4 apples.

ADULT & CHILD Measure the brown sugar or syrup. Distribute the sugar or syrup equally inside each of the 4 apples.

ADULT Place in the preheated oven and bake about 15 to 20 minutes, or until the apples are very soft inside and the peels are very shiny. Serve with a dollop of crème fraîche or sour cream, if desired.

PREP TIME	COOK TIME	YIELD
5 minutes	15 to 20 minutes	4 to 6 servings

{ DAY 7 } Understand Food Marketing Deception

UNLESS YOU LIVE ON ANOTHER PLANET, you cannot avoid the messages commercial food companies aim at your kids. According to the Center for Science in the Public Interest, food and beverage companies spend billions of dollars annually to market their products to children. Even two-year-olds are targets.

The Institute of Medicine published in 2006 the most comprehensive review of the scientific evidence of the influence of food marketing on what children prefer to eat and drink. Sadly, most of what is marketed to children are sweets, soft drinks, salty snacks, and fast foods that increase their risk of obesity. Obese children are more likely to become obese adults, with an increased risk of developing diabetes and other chronic diseases.

How can parents fight back against the advertisers who are enticing our kids? We recommend undermining the efforts of these marketers. This may be the best way to shield our children from unhealthy eating habits.

playing food detective is both fun and educational

Our "Food Detective" game helps children connect the dots so they learn to be suspicious of packaged food and not trust appearances. Inspired by the

"Don't Buy It" web page at www.pbs.org, we developed this game and have used it successfully for many years in schools and with our own children. We undermine the advertisers when, for instance, we show kids that strawberries may appear on the label of a fruit juice that looks so delicious, but *no* strawberries are in the juice—only artificial flavors and sugars! Children may still like to drink the liquid, but at least they understand it's artificial, closer to candy than real food provided by nature.

To play this game, choose any packaged food designed to appeal especially to children—snacks, cereal, fruit drinks. Ask questions about the food and discuss their answers. This deductive process is a fun way to have a conversation about what they eat and how marketing pros trick them into making unhealthy choices. Here are some questions to spark discussion:

1. What pictures are on the package?
2. What words and images are used to attract your attention?
3. How do they make the food appealing?

Ask questions about the food and discuss their answers. This deductive process is a fun way to have a conversation about what they eat and how marketing pros trick them into making unhealthy choices.

4. Who is this item targeted to? Analyze the colors, fonts, and any cartoon characters or people pictured using the item.

5. Are toys or prizes offered? Are they actually inside?

6. Do the pictures on the package represent what is actually inside the box?

7. What foods pictured on the package are *not* mentioned in the ingredients list?

8. Is the food pictured on the package the main ingredient?

9. Do you think this product is nutritious? Why or why not? How can you be sure?

10. How do food marketers try to convince you to buy their product?

use food marketers' tactics to your advantage

By now you are purchasing more whole foods and serving more of them to your family. Hopefully you are planning meals seasonally and considering some new recipe concepts. You've taken the entire family on a farmers' market excursion. However, you're probably getting some resistance from your family, too, as you work hard to provide healthier meals. To counteract this resistance, let's learn more about the tactics food marketers use to entice your children and *use them to your advantage*.

The following chart reviews some of the marketers' tactics in the left column. On the right, we show you how to use the same tactics to win over your kids to healthy choices. If you think doing this is a lot of effort, keep in mind that marketers have spent billions on it—they know it works!

7 savvy tactics stolen from food marketers to get your kids to eat more veggies

marketing tactic	use it to encourage healthy food choices
attractiveness colorful shapes and images (bright colors with cartoon characters, animals)	Contrast colors in a dish, such as stir-fry or salad, to make it more visually tempting. Set a beautiful or fun table. Go ahead and use colorful cartoon character plates, but only to introduce new and healthy recipes. Put superhero figures in lunch boxes to "guard" kids' favorite healthy foods.
bribery offering toys with purchase (toys in cereal boxes or with fast foods)	Bribery works, but use it at your discretion with healthy foods. Never use dessert as a reward. Maybe offer to play endless Monopoly or other game.
promise the world using health claims and superheroes to convince kids they will be smarter, cooler, and more popular	Similarly, we associate stories about foods when we introduce traditional recipes in our programs. Many cultures incorporate food into their mythology. Example: Thai children thank the "Rice Mother" at every meal because "food" in Thai is synonymous with rice.
vocabulary amazing, enticing, and memorable names create higher expectations ("lucky charms")	Lynn names recipes after friends and family: "Linda's Carrot Cake" and "Jimmy's Favorite Macaroni." Kids are creative; they'll rename all your recipes for you. We also ask children to describe the sensations of the food they experience—they love to use their imaginations.
music playing music to put you in a good mood and make you form pleasant associations with supermarkets and fast food restaurants	Mercedes plays music her children like while cooking good food. This encourages them to hang out in the kitchen, to associate good food with their favorite songs, and to clean up the kitchen after meals.
access to fun providing a playground, such as at mcdonald's, to attract families, making it easy on parents	Bring healthy snacks or a picnic lunch to a park with a playground. Let kids play arts and crafts in your kitchen while you cook and they munch on veggies.
health claims claiming to support your health	Health claims work! Children like to know how nutrients protect them and help their bodies grow. Mercedes' son liked to associate every fruit and veggie with an arsenal of protection: garlic gave him tanks, pomegranates provided grenades, and citrus fruits made up the infantry.

rhubarb and blueberry muffins

The streusel topping on these muffins makes them extra delicious. You can switch up the fruit inside, but keep it colorful.

¼ cup (55 g) butter, softened

1½ cups (340 g) packed brown sugar

1 egg

3 stalks rhubarb, 10 inches (25.4 cm) long each

2 cups (240 g) flour

1 teaspoon baking soda

½ teaspoon salt

1 cup (230 g) plain yogurt

¾ cup (109 g) blueberries

½ cup (60 g) walnuts

½ cup (100 g) granulated sugar

1 tablespoon (7 g) ground cinnamon

2 tablespoons (28 g) butter

ADDITIONAL COOKING EQUIPMENT:
Electric mixer, muffin tin

NOTE: *Children should use plastic or table knives for all child steps that require cutting or chopping.*

ADULT Preheat oven to 350°F (180°C, or gas mark 4).

ADULT & CHILD Measure the ¼ cup (55 g) butter and brown sugar into a mixing bowl. Beat with electric mixer or wooden spoon until creamy.

ADULT & CHILD Crack the egg on edge of a bowl; with two thumbs in the crack, the child can separate the halves and drop the egg into the bowl. Beat until fully incorporated.

CHILD Cut the rhubarb into ½-inch (13 mm)-long pieces.

ADULT & CHILD Measure the flour, baking soda, and salt. Mix into the butter mixture just until all the dry ingredients are moistened. Measure and add the yogurt, and mix until everything is well incorporated. Measure the blueberries. Add the rhubarb and blueberries and mix well.

ADULT & CHILD Place paper muffin cups in muffin tin. Spoon mixture into cups, making sure batter fills cups no more than two-thirds full.

ADULT Chop the walnuts coarsely, and put into a bowl.

CHILD Measure the granulated sugar and cinnamon and add to the walnuts.

ADULT Melt the 2 tablespoons (28 g) butter in a small saucepan over low heat, or in the microwave. Pour over the sugar, cinnamon, and walnuts.

ADULT & CHILD Mix well with a wooden spoon. Spoon a teaspoon of topping over the muffins.

ADULT Bake muffins in preheated oven about 20 minutes, or until a toothpick inserted in a muffin comes out clean. Serve warm or store for three days in an airtight container.

PREP TIME	COOK TIME	YIELD
15 minutes	20 minutes	12 to 18 muffins

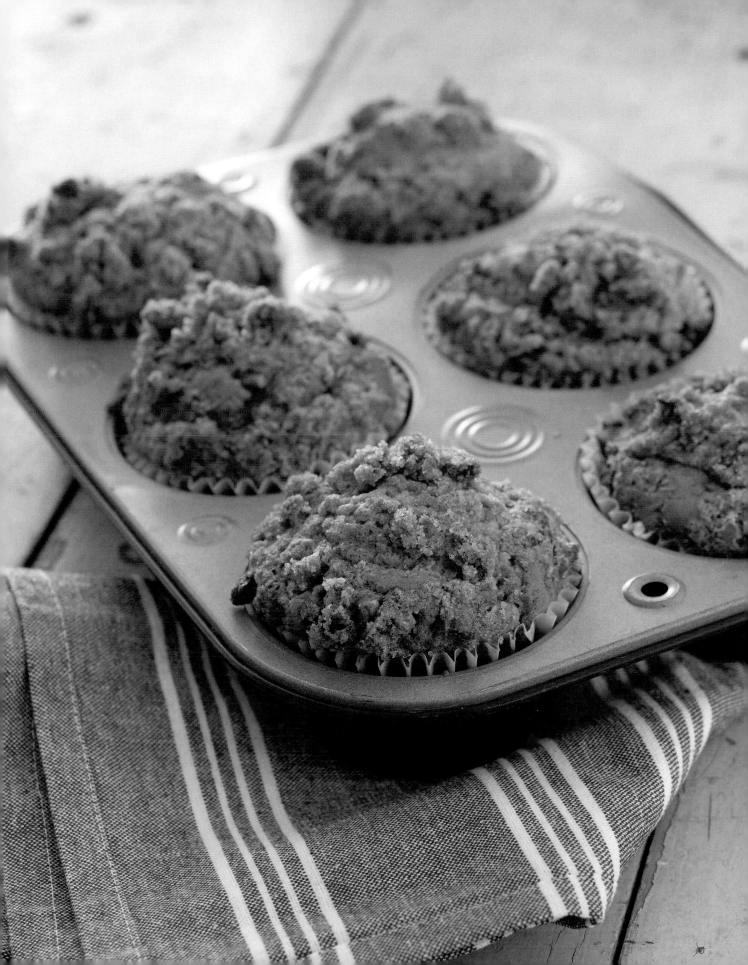

{ DAY 7 }

summer stone fruit salad

A celebration of summer tree fruit, this recipe gives you a great reason to invest in a cherry pitter. Substitute other colorful fruit during different seasons.

3 sprigs fresh mint

3 tablespoons (45 g) turbinado raw sugar

4 peaches (ideally 2 white, 2 yellow)

4 apricots

3 plums

½ pound (225 g) cherries, pitted (optional)

½ lime

ADDITIONAL COOKING EQUIPMENT:
Food processor

NOTE: *Children should use plastic or table knives for all child steps that require cutting or chopping.*

CHILD Separate mint leaves from stems.

ADULT & CHILD Help measure the sugar. Using a food processor, grind the mint leaves and sugar until fine. Transfer to a large mixing bowl.

ADULT Cut the peaches, apricots, and plums in half; remove pits.

CHILD Help slice the fruit halves into 6 to 8 even slices. Add to mixing bowl with the mint and sugar.

ADULT & CHILD Cut the pitted cherries in half and add to the mixing bowl, if using. Squeeze lime half over all of the fruit.

CHILD Mix thoroughly and chill for 10 minutes before serving.

PREP TIME
15 minutes

YIELD
8 to 10 servings

{ DAY 8 } Avoid Additives

FOR THOUSANDS OF YEARS, people have been drying, salting, freezing, pickling, and otherwise preserving and processing foods to make them last longer. But in recent decades, parents have found themselves in a whole other ballgame. Many of today's foods contain all sorts of additives to extend their shelf life. Some food products are made almost entirely of synthetic ingredients.

Of course you don't intentionally opt to include a portion of sodium nitrate, artificial sweeteners, emulsifiers, and artificial coloring in your children's lunches or your family's dinner. But by shopping mindlessly you can overload your family with potentially harmful ingredients that can adversely affect their health and behavior. And what children eat in their early years can have an impact on their food preferences for life.

Yes, the U.S. Food and Drug Administration considers many additives safe and allows manufacturers to put them in our food. It can take decades of research and study to show that certain ingredients are harmful. Why take a chance when your children's health is at stake? You have a choice. When shopping for peanut butter, bread, tomato sauce, or any other packaged food, you can buy a pure, unadulterated product or bring home something loaded with additives.

shop mindfully so you make healthy choices

Shopping mindfully may confuse you and seem awfully time consuming, especially in the beginning. You may even feel a bit overwhelmed at times. Reading all those labels and analyzing all those ingredients can seem daunting. Even minimally processed food—air-popped corn, tofu, canned beans

and tomatoes—require scrutiny.

But when you shop carefully for packaged foods, you help your family become healthy for life. And it does get easier over time as you learn what to look for. It just takes a little practice. Shopping mindfully also tells food companies that there are shoppers like you who demand high quality. Consumer pressure has caused many companies to produce more health-conscious foods in recent years.

six smart steps to mindful shopping

You can determine a product's quality simply by reading the ingredients list. However, don't burn yourself out by trying to do everything perfectly right away. Approach shopping mindfully as a project done over a period of weeks or even months. Before long, you'll develop a routine that makes the process much quicker and easier. Here are six steps to mindful shopping:

1. Make a list of the packaged foods you buy most frequently.
2. Choose one packaged food at a time to analyze.
3. Ignore the pictures, messages, and health claims on the package.
4. Focus exclusively on the ingredients list, which can sometimes be printed in really small letters or positioned in dark, hard-to-find places.

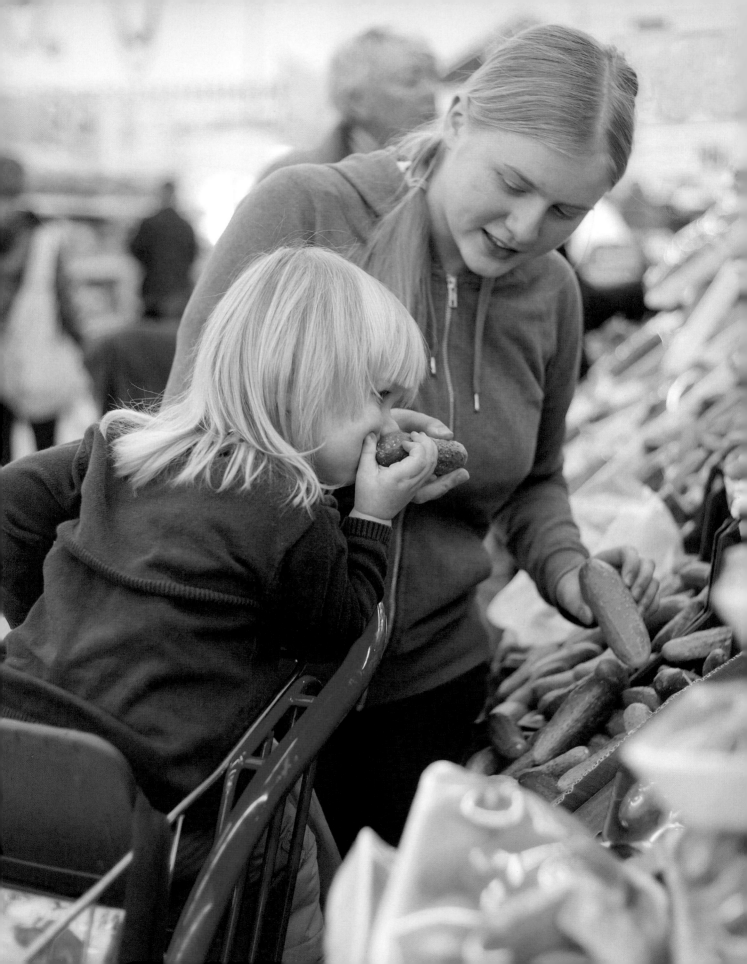

learn about chemical additives

The Chemical Cuisine glossary of food additives on the website of the Center for Science in the Public Interest is the best place to clarify unintelligible ingredients. Visit www.cspinet.org/reports/chemcuisine.htm for information—and it now offers a mobile app!

5. Look at the order of ingredients: By law, ingredients must be listed in descending order by weight. That means the first ingredients are the main ingredients. Unfortunately, food companies are not obliged to tell you how much of each ingredient is included. But consider this: If, for example, you're paying for blueberry juice, why buy a brand that has apple juice listed as the first ingredient?

6. Scrutinize the ingredients list for unnecessary additives, such as monoglycerides, calcium propionate, or calcium sulfate. Your reference should be homemade food. For example, if you baked bread at home, it would contain only flour, water, yeast, and maybe salt. Anything else you see listed on packaged bread is a chemical added for the company's convenience and to extend shelf life. The same is true of breakfast cereals. If you made oatmeal from whole grain, it would only include oats and water, plus whatever you use to flavor it such as milk or honey. But instant oatmeal and packaged cereals contain long lists of ingredients.

distinguish among common additives to determine their value

Packaged foods often contain added vitamins, fiber, and sugars:

♡ **vitamins:** These are added to white flours to make up for what's lost in the refining process, such as ascorbic acid (vitamin C), niacinamide, iron, pyridoxine hydrochloride (vitamin B6), riboflavin (vitamin B2), vitamin A, palmitate, thiamine hydrochloride (vitamin B1), folic acid.

♡ **sugars:** These are added to many packaged foods and can contribute to obesity. They go by many different names, such as molasses, corn syrup, high fructose corn syrup, invert sugar, or any sweetener ending with -ose.

♡ **dietary fiber:** A common health claim on food products, dietary fibers may include inulin, wheat dextrin, and methylcellulose. You and your family will get all the fiber you need by eating more legumes, whole grains, fruit, and vegetables.

get started

Learn to understand nutrition labels on packaged products:

♡ Compare two (or more) different brands of a favorite product, such as peanut butter, to determine what ingredients each contains. Does one have more additives than the other?

♡ Look carefully at the Nutrition Facts on labels for both brands to determine which is the healthier choice. What makes it healthier?

♡ Consider the serving size and the number of calories in each serving.

♡ How are the calories derived? Do they come from nutrients and the principal food (peanuts), or do they come from added sugars and unhealthy fats?

♡ Explain to your children how to choose a quality peanut butter.

♡ Walk your children through the process so they understand what to look for.

♡ Do a blind tasting with your kids, comparing a pure brand of peanut butter against a more adulterated one.

arugula and peach salad

When fruit is cooked in butter and browned, their sugars become concentrated. Dropped into the greens in this salad, these bursts of warm juicy flavor provide a fabulous contrast with spicy arugula.

1 pound (455 g) arugula, washed very thoroughly

2 medium peaches

1 tablespoon (14 g) butter

Nuts or sunflower seeds (optional)

1 tablespoon (15 ml) olive oil

1 teaspoon rice or cider vinegar

Salt and pepper

NOTE: *Children should use plastic or table knives for all child steps that require cutting or chopping.*

ADULT & CHILD Place the arugula in a serving bowl.

ADULT Cut the peaches in half; remove the pits.

ADULT & CHILD Slice the peaches into segments about ½ inch (13 mm) thick.

ADULT Melt the butter in a small skillet over medium heat. Reduce heat to low and add the peaches. Cook and stir for about 8 minutes, or until peaches are slightly caramelized or browned.

ADULT & CHILD Add peach slices to the serving bowl. Add nuts or seeds and mix well.

ADULT & CHILD Measure the olive oil and vinegar. Pour each over the salad and mix well (try to keep all the peaches from falling to the bottom). Season to taste with salt and pepper.

PREP TIME	COOK TIME	YIELD
5 minutes	8 minutes	4 to 6 servings

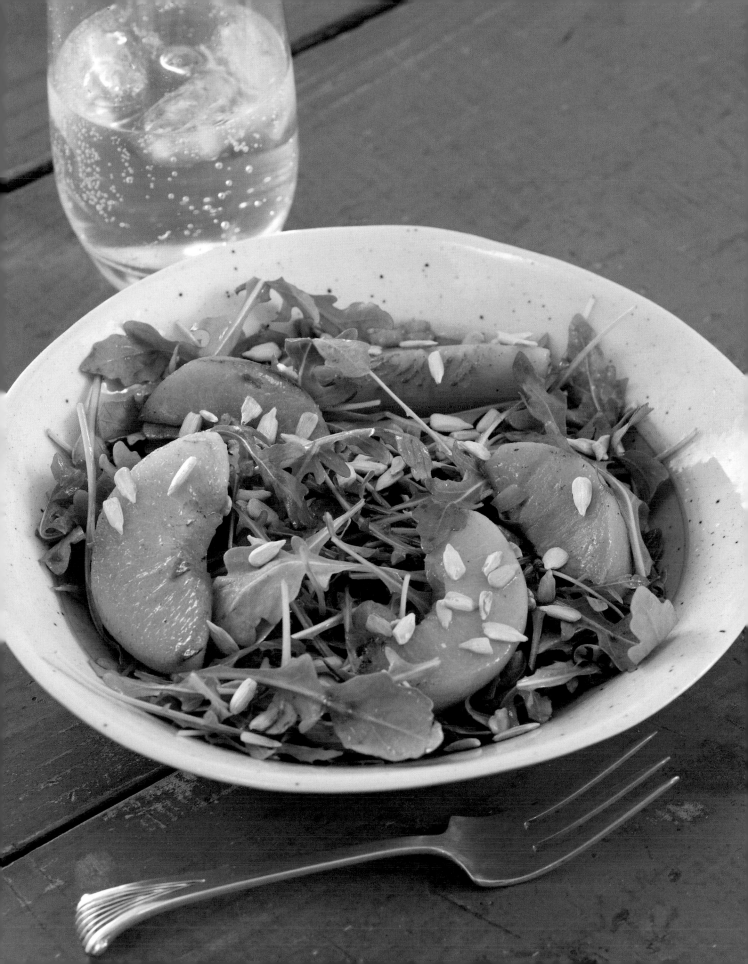

tuscan bean soup

One of the most popular recipes in our FamilyCook repertoire, this soup is a hit with all ages. Although you can use any combination of greens, this particular blend gives just the right balance of sweet and bitter.

1 medium onion

2 cloves garlic

2 tablespoons (30 ml) olive oil

½ bunch kale

½ bunch broccoli rabe

2 cans (14 ounces, or 397 g) white cannellini beans

1 can (28 ounces, or 794 g) whole tomatoes

4 cups (946 ml) chicken broth

3 sprigs fresh thyme

Kosher salt and freshly ground pepper

1 loaf (16 ounces, or 455 g) Italian bread

NOTE: *Children should use plastic or table knives for all child steps that require cutting or chopping.*

ADULT Slice the onion.

CHILD Chop the onion into small pieces.

ADULT Smash the garlic with the flat side of the chef's knife to remove the peel and slice.

ADULT Heat a large stockpot over medium heat. Add olive oil. When the oil is hot, add the chopped onion and reduce the heat to low. Cook, stirring occasionally, about 10 minutes, or until onions are translucent.

CHILD Meanwhile, help chop the garlic slices and add to the onion. Help stir for three minutes or until lightly browned or onions are ready, using oven mitts to protect hands from heat.

CHILD While the onions are cooking, help tear up the kale and broccoli rabe.

ADULT Add the greens to the stockpot, increase heat to medium, and stir the greens until they wilt.

CHILD Help open the cans of beans and tomatoes with a can opener.

CHILD With clean hands, squeeze the tomatoes into the stockpot.

ADULT Drain and rinse the beans in a colander. Add to the stockpot and bring to simmer, cooking 5 more minutes.

CHILD Help stir while adult adds the chicken broth (using oven mitts to protect hands while stirring).

CHILD Pluck the thyme leaves from their stems. Add to the pot.

ADULT Season to taste with salt and freshly ground pepper.

ADULT Cook an additional 10 minutes and serve with Italian bread.

PREP TIME	COOK TIME	YIELD
10 minutes	25 minutes	4 servings

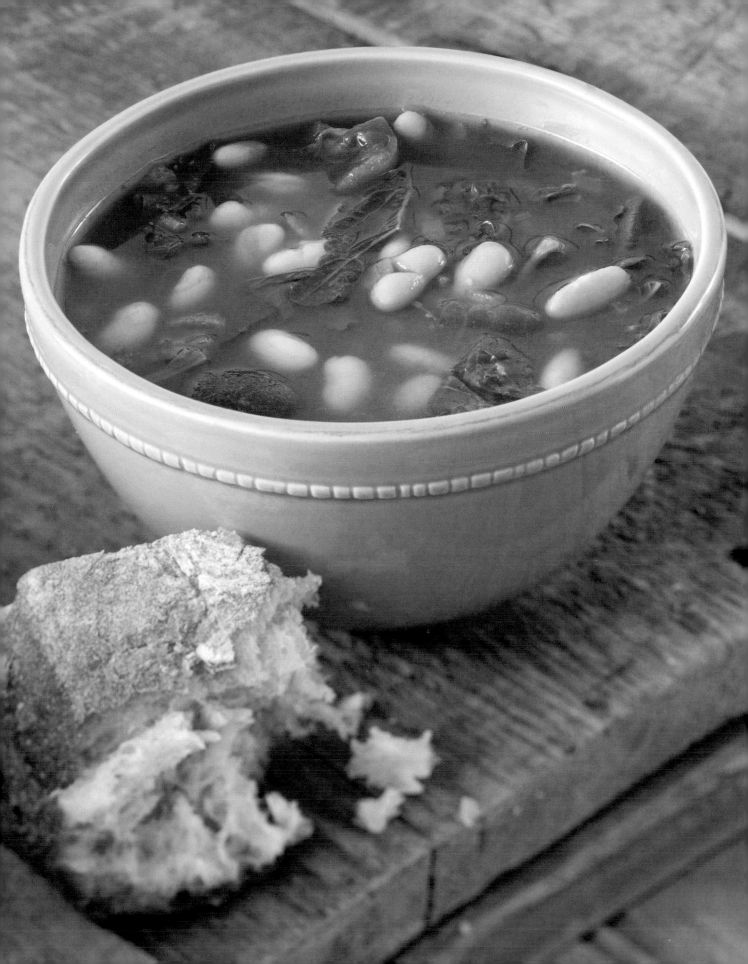

PART 3

IMPROVE YOUR SKILLS AS COOK AND NOURISHER

{ DAY 9 } Make Your Kitchen a Family Retreat

COOKING MEALS TOGETHER gives you a wonderful opportunity to bond with your children. Even though your hands may be occupied, you can give kids your attention and enjoy their company. It's the ideal time to transmit your culture, stories, and fond memories about food. And the seductive aromas reel them in.

Over the past few decades, many kitchens have become mere heat-and-serve environments, where prepared foods are warmed up in the microwave. This deprives our children of the sensory experiences of cooking whole foods in their natural state. Nor do kids get to witness meals being prepared with love. Worse still, our role as nourishers is taken over by impersonal sources: food corporations and fast-food restaurants.

Lynn grew up in the Chicago suburbs and remembers hanging out with her mom in the kitchen when she was a girl. As they chatted, Lynn happily nibbled the tasty food. Mesmerized, she watched as her mom poured steaming olive-green spinach linguine into a colander. She couldn't resist swooping down to grab a strand. She vividly remembers the aromas of garlic, tomatoes, peppers, pungent fresh parsley and basil, and delicate shrimp and scallops when her mother cooked eye-poppingly colorful cioppino, an Italian seafood stew. Mother

> **MISSION FOR THE DAY**
>
> Make your kitchen a welcoming place for the whole family.

and daughter connected richly as Lynn shadowed her mom's every move.

Years later, Lynn discovered that we learn best through our senses. She realized that her sensory experiences with food in her youth formed her love for home-cooked meals made from fresh ingredients. Such sensory experiences will empower your own children later in their lives, too. When the kitchen is alive, children connect deeply with real food in all its stages, from raw to ready to eat. Even if your child does not become interested in cooking, just being exposed to the wonderful smells and sounds of cooking in your kitchen will be an essential part of his or her food education.

As FamilyCook Productions evolved, we sought to create sensory references for the families we taught. We successfully turned the classroom into a magical kitchen where children cooked together, fascinated by what they prepared and ate. The experience made indelible impressions on these youngsters.

Cook at home and you'll show your children how fresh ingredients are transformed into healthy meals. You'll help them connect more deeply with the role meals play in your family life. This emotional hook will help you stick with your goals even when you feel pressed for time.

Cooking family meals at home today can seem like an uphill battle for many families. You don't need a huge space and all the latest appliances to make your kitchen an appealing place to cook together. Even a cramped urban nook can become a welcoming spot where you and your kids will want to spend time making healthy family meals.

On Day 1, we suggested making small changes in your kitchen so you would be more comfortable there. Now it's time to entice the rest of your family to join you.

design your kitchen to tantalize all five senses

You don't need to call an architect or spend a lot of money revamping your kitchen. Simply consider how you can make it an inviting family retreat. How can you organize the space so you have adequate room to cook and so your children can watch you? What adjustments can you make so your kitchen tantalizes all the senses of anyone who enters? Here are some suggestions:

- ♡ **sights:** Display fruits and vegetables of every color and shape in bowls or on platters. Don't hide everything away in the refrigerator.
- ♡ **aromas:** Collect and use many different types of seasonings: sweet floral honey, spicy chile peppers, heady aromatic curries, tangy vinegars. When you cook our international recipes, new scents will permeate the air.
- ♡ **sounds:** The sounds of water running, your knife chopping veggies, tools and pots clanging, the mortar and pestle grinding, and appliances whirring let your family know that delicious food is on the way.

- ♡ **textures:** Revel in the many and varied textures of the food you prepare: hard and moist root veggies, tickly and prickly tubers, fuzzy kiwis, squirty plums, sticky peaches. Laugh about these sensations as you share them with your children.
- ♡ **flavors:** Make it a game to describe the taste of a recipe's ingredients in the most intriguing way. Use a variety of words: sweet, tart, puckery sour, salty, bitter, spicy, peachy, cucumberish, tomatoey. Let kids make up their own descriptions—the more unique and humorous, the better.

As you repeatedly expose children to the delicious sensory experiences involved with food preparation, you encourage them to spend more time in the family kitchen. You evoke in them a greater appreciation of food. And you help them understand why it's important to take time to make healthy meals—now and when they have kitchens of their own in the future.

🕐 get started

Make your kitchen a place where your kids want to hang out:

- ♡ When you are cooking meals, invite them in to enjoy a snack or do their homework.
- ♡ Chat with them about something they enjoy— this is not a time to have serious discussions.
- ♡ Keep a step stool handy so very young helpers can reach the counter or the stove for a supervised stir.
- ♡ Arrange chairs or stools near the table or counter so kids can spend time helping with cooking tasks, doing homework, or other projects.
- ♡ Lay out paper and pens—all that sensory exposure could inspire some lovely artwork to decorate your kitchen.

wild rice salad

There is something almost addictive about the flavor combinations in this salad. It's also nearly seasonless, so you can make it anytime.

1 cup (160 g) wild rice, or a combo of wild and other rice

2 cups (475 ml) water

¼ teaspoon salt

1 cup (120 g) walnuts

1 celery rib

4 scallions

¾ cup (110 g) raisins

1 medium apple (Granny Smith or other tart variety)

1 lemon

3 tablespoons (45 ml) freshly squeezed lemon juice

½ teaspoon salt

⅓ cup (80 ml) olive oil

Freshly ground black pepper

ADDITIONAL COOKING EQUIPMENT: Box grater, apple corer and segmenter

NOTE: *Children should use plastic or table knives for all child steps that require cutting or chopping.*

ADULT Rinse rice in a strainer under cold water. Place rice in a medium saucepan along with the water and the ¼ teaspoon salt. Cover, bring to a boil, and reduce the heat to simmer. Cook 50 minutes, or until the rice is tender and all the water has been absorbed. You may need to add more water to get the rice to a nice tender consistency. (When fully cooked, the kernels will burst slightly and have a tender texture.)

ADULT & CHILD Chop the walnuts and thinly slice celery and scallions. Add to a large mixing bowl.

CHILD Help measure raisins and add to the bowl.

ADULT Core and segment the apple. Slice each of the 8 segments into 2 slices.

CHILD Help chop the apples into tiny dice. Add to the mixing bowl.

ADULT & CHILD Grate the lemon rind with the box grater. Let young children help by holding the end of the lemon while you hold their hands and help them go up and down once or twice. Older children can do this independently.

ADULT Add rind to the bowl. Cut the lemon in half to be squeezed.

CHILD Help squeeze and measure the lemon juice, and measure the ½ teaspoon salt, olive oil, and pepper. Place all in a jar with a tight-fitting lid. Place lid on jar and shake to mix well.

ADULT When rice is done, let cool, then add to the bowl. Pour on the lemon juice–olive oil dressing to taste and toss well. Chill for 10 to 15 minutes before serving.

PREP TIME	YIELD
1 hour	8 servings

poached pears in red wine

The poaching liquid becomes a delectable and fragrant sauce you'll love. If you have some left over, keep it for drizzling over ice cream or cheese for a lovely contrast of flavors.

6 Bosc pears with stems, or other varieties

2 cups (475 ml) red wine

½ cup (100 g) sugar

1 lemon

1 cinnamon stick

3 whole cloves

1 teaspoon vanilla extract

NOTE: *Children should use plastic or table knives for all child steps that require cutting or chopping.*

tip

May be prepared a day in advance and chilled and then served at room temperature.

ADULT Peel and core the pears. Cut into quarters.

CHILD Help measure the wine and sugar.

ADULT Place the pears in a large saucepan, and add the wine and sugar.

ADULT Peel the lemon and slice the peel into very thin julienne strips. Reserve the peeled lemon for another use.

ADULT & CHILD Add the lemon peel to the saucepan. Add the cinnamon stick and cloves. Measure and add the vanilla.

ADULT Bring liquid to a boil over medium-high heat, then turn heat to low and simmer for 5 to 10 minutes, or until pears are tender. Transfer the pears and the lemon peel to a serving dish.

ADULT Bring the liquid in the saucepan to a boil once again. Reduce liquid by half, or until it becomes syrupy. Pour the sauce over the pears. Cool and serve warm or at room temperature.

PREP TIME	COOK TIME	YIELD
20 minutes	15 minutes	6 servings

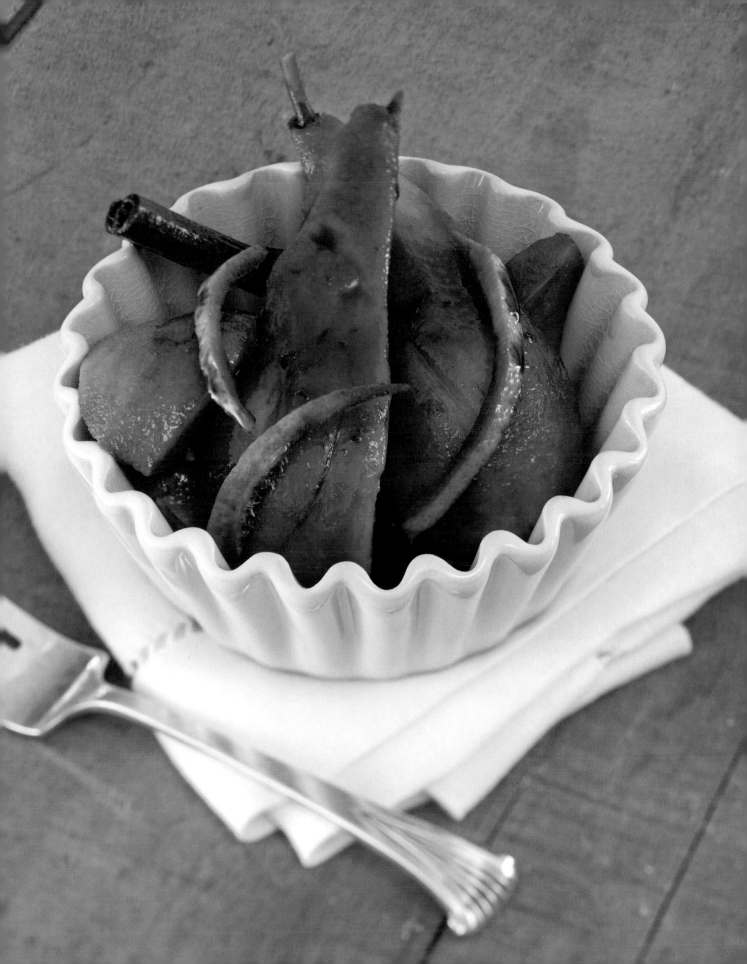

farm vegetable quiche

Your family will enjoy reinventing this satisfying recipe concept using their favorite vegetables and cheese combinations. If you're pressed for time, you can cheat and use a prepared pie crust. Just keep some in your freezer for such emergencies.

1 small onion, or 2 large leeks

2 tablespoons (28 g) butter

1 pound (455 g) Swiss chard or other greens

1/3 bunch fresh dill or basil, rinsed and dried

3 eggs

1 cup (235 ml) milk

1/2 cup (120 ml) cream

2/3 cup (113 g) cheese (goat, cow, or combination)

Kosher salt and freshly ground pepper

1 pie shell, thawed

NOTE: *Children should use plastic or table knives for all child steps that require cutting or chopping.*

tips

- Vary vegetables based on the season.
- Be sure to blanch or sauté the vegetable(s) you choose.
- Try different cheeses— gruyere, fontina, pecorino.

ADULT Preheat oven to 350°F (180°C, or gas mark 4). Slice the onion or leeks.

ADULT Heat the butter in a small skillet, add the onions, and reduce heat. Cook about 10 minutes, or until translucent.

CHILD Help tear or chop the chard.

ADULT Fill a medium saucepan halfway with water and bring to a boil. Blanch the greens in boiling water, about 2 minutes. Drain in a colander.

CHILD Help chop the fresh dill or snip with scissors. Set aside.

ADULT & CHILD In a large mixing bowl, crack the eggs on edge of a bowl; with two thumbs in the crack, the child can separate the halves and drop the eggs into the bowl. Beat the eggs with a whisk.

ADULT In a mixing bowl, combine the softened onions with the chard and dill. Mix well.

ADULT & CHILD Measure the milk and cream, add to the beaten eggs, and mix well. Crumble the cheese into the egg mixture. Season with salt and pepper.

ADULT & CHILD Add the chard mixture to the pie shell, distributing evenly. Pour the egg and cheese mixture on top.

ADULT Bake for about 40 minutes, or until the custard is set.

PREP TIME	COOK TIME	YIELD
15 minutes	40 minutes	6 servings

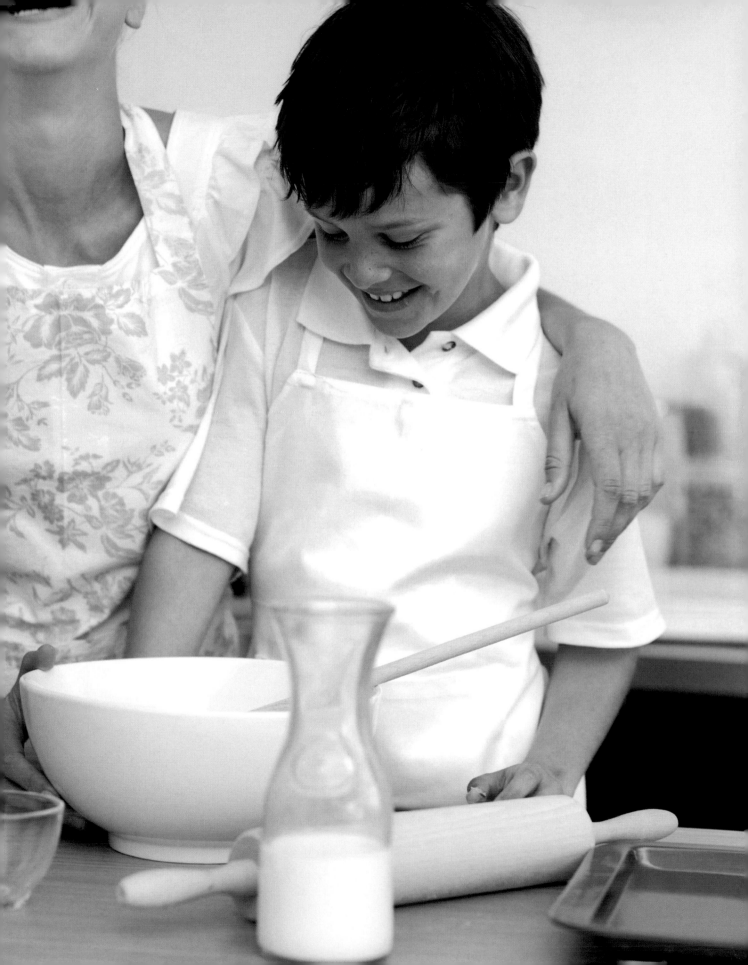

{DAY 10} Own Your Role as Nourisher

YOU'VE COME THIS FAR because you are a nourisher. You understand that the quality and healthfulness of the food you provide will have an impact on your family's long-term health. By now your efforts have yielded some victories and surprises. But likely you've experienced some setbacks, too. What can be more discouraging than making a beautiful seasonal recipe, only to have your children take one look and refuse to eat it—especially after you've invested precious time and money on quality ingredients? Now you're worried that your children are starving, and yet they won't eat.

At such times you may feel tempted to give up and revert to serving meals you know they will eat but aren't as nutritious. We are not going to lie; we understand this transition is not easy. However, your frustration is totally normal. After years of receiving external pressures from food marketers, peers, and others, it will take a while for you and your family to make these big changes. Don't be discouraged. We'll offer some field-tested guidance to set you and your family up for success.

be persistent and consistent to win kids over to healthy eating

The only way your family can come to enjoy a balanced diet is to be exposed day after day to meals that contain necessary nutrients from a variety of healthy foods. All our recipes are well balanced and should provide enough food to satisfy hunger. They

MISSION FOR THE DAY

Strategize the best routine for your family's meals and snack times.

include a wide range of whole and minimally processed foods—plenty of fruits and vegetables, whole grains, and plant-based proteins—so both adults and children can eat well and maintain healthy weights. This new diet provides all five essential nutrients: vitamins, minerals, carbohydrates, proteins, and fats (those which occur naturally in real food), as well as phytochemicals and fiber. Your family's palates and preferences will adapt to these fresh flavors as they become familiar with new foods. That's why your perseverance is so important.

When you serve something new, be sure to also offer foods that you are confident your family will eat. If they don't react enthusiastically to a new recipe, explain that you are only asking them to try it. Never force a child to eat something, and don't make it a big deal that you are disappointed. Rather, say with assurance, "I'm sure you'll grow to like it." Acknowledge that as children grow they will discover that their tastes change. In the meantime, the food your children reject can become a nice lunch for you to take to work the next day.

Keep on serving those rejected foods, trying different ways to prepare and serve them. By exploring new foods again and again, your children will become accustomed to experimenting and be happily surprised when they find that some taste good. You never know when they'll decide to eat a second helping of a food they once claimed they hated.

schedule regular meals and snacks to ensure metabolic rhythm

Maintaining a structure for family meals and snacks can also help you succeed as a nourisher. A regular eating schedule promotes a metabolic rhythm and prevents hunger peaks that can lead to overeating. Ellyn Satter, registered dietitian, author, and a leading authority on feeding children, created a "Division of Responsibility in Feeding" concept that has helped parents understand their duties and become more confident nourishers.

Satter's research has shown that parents who provide regular sit-down meals achieve positive results in their children's eating behaviors over time. Children learn to eat the food their parents eat and eventually begin to model their parents' table manners. Given time, children will eat the amount they need and make food choices that will balance their nutritional needs.

make sure adolescents get the nutrition they need for optimal growth

Eating healthy is essential at all ages and stages of life to promote optimal growth and well-being, and to prevent diet-related diseases. Adolescence is the trickiest stage. It's the second-fastest growth stage, next to infancy. Over this period of several years, children gain 20 percent of their adult height, 50 percent of their adult weight, and 40 percent of their adult skeletal mass. Poor nutrition can put this growth at risk.

Adolescents are hungrier and need more calories than younger children; some very active teens may need to eat up to 3,000 calories a day, or even more if they play vigorous sports. Make sure they get plenty of calcium and vitamin D, too, to ensure healthy bone development. Although kids need a nutritious diet to grow to their full potential, they probably won't make it easy for you. During this period they are growing more independent, are searching for their identity, and are hyper concerned with appearance and peer acceptance. As a result, their eating behavior, weight, and nutritional status may be affected.

The good news is, most adolescents are more adventurous than younger children about exploring new foods—but they usually want to explore on their own. This can be a good time to introduce new foods to them in a celebratory, fun way. It is also an ideal time to encourage them to cook recipes by themselves. You know your teenagers best. What roles will they embrace in planning and cooking family meals? Ask them. Maybe he'd like to help with menu planning and shopping, or be in charge of preparing dinner one night a week. Maybe she prefers to be the salad master every night. Let them decide how they can best contribute.

⏱ get started

Now that you're more confident in your role of nourisher, here are some tips to help you stay motivated and on track:

- ♡ Determine the best times to schedule meals and snacks.
- ♡ Try to synchronize schedules so the entire family sits down to eat a meal together at least once a day—we're just saying *try*.
- ♡ Visit the American Academy of Pediatrics' website www.healthychildren.org for guidance on nutritional needs for all ages.

danielle's fiber-rich banana bread

Friend and colleague Danielle O'Connell is a fantastic wellness practitioner, mom, and home cook. Her vegan banana bread amazed Lynn, who prefers its delicious nutty flavor and interesting texture to any other banana bread recipe.

4 ripe bananas

⅓ cup (80 ml) canola oil

½ cup (100 g) sugar

½ cup (125 g) applesauce

1½ teaspoon vanilla extract

4 tablespoons (48 g) ground flaxseeds

1 teaspoon baking soda

Pinch of salt

2 tablespoons (30 ml) agave nectar

1½ cup (188 g) whole wheat flour

ADDITIONAL COOKING EQUIPMENT:
9 x 5 x 3-inch (23 x 13 x 7.5 cm) loaf pan, coffee grinder (optional)

NOTE: *Children should use plastic or table knives for all child steps that require cutting or chopping.*

ADULT Preheat the oven to 350°F (180°C, or gas mark 4).

ADULT & CHILD Peel the bananas and mash with a fork. Place in a large mixing bowl.

ADULT & CHILD Measure the oil. Mix the oil into the mashed bananas with a wooden spoon.

ADULT & CHILD Measure the sugar, applesauce, and vanilla. Add to the bowl.

ADULT & CHILD Measure the ground flaxseeds, baking soda, and salt and add to the mixture. Measure and add agave nectar.

ADULT & CHILD Measure and add the flour. Stir until ingredients are well incorporated. Pour into a greased 9 x 5 x 3-inch (23 x 13 x 7.5 cm) loaf pan.

ADULT Bake 50 to 60 minutes, or until the top springs back when slightly depressed. Cool on a rack.

tip

If you don't have a spice grinder, grind the flaxseeds in a coffee grinder.

PREP TIME	COOK TIME	YIELD
15 minutes	50 to 60 minutes	1 loaf

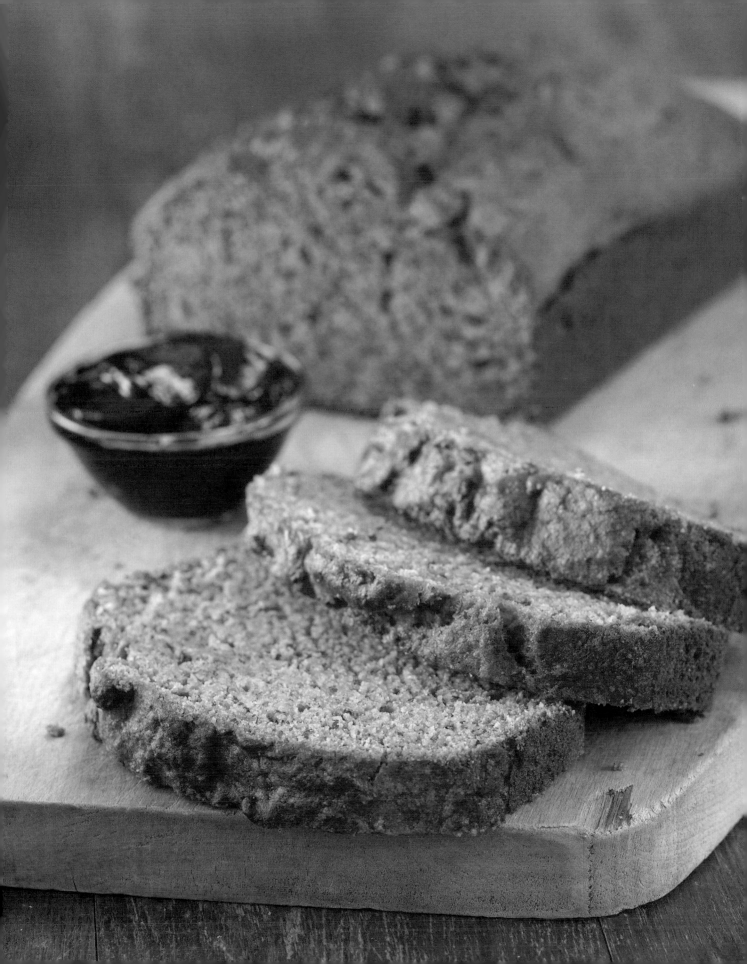

ten-minute yogurt-cucumber soup

Most cucumber soups require cooking, but this recipe doesn't and can be made in minutes. It's delicious and refreshing on a hot summer day and festive when garnished with edible flower petals (pansy, geranium, or nasturtium) from your garden. Lynn's personal favorite are borage flowers.

2 cloves garlic

¼ to ½ red onion

½ green bell pepper

1 handful assorted fresh herbs (dill, parsley, mint, basil)

2 cucumbers

1 cup (235 ml) water, divided

2 cups (475 ml) whole milk or low-fat yogurt

Salt and pepper

Edible flower petals (pansy, geranium, nasturtium, borage) for garnish (optional)

ADDITIONAL COOKING EQUIPMENT: Electric stand blender or immersion blender, tall cylindrical container

NOTE: *Children should use plastic or table knives for all child steps that require cutting or chopping.*

ADULT Smash the garlic with the flat side of chef's knife to remove peel. Slice the garlic, onion, and bell pepper in slices.

CHILD Snip the herbs and set aside. Cut the garlic, onion, and bell pepper into smaller pieces.

ADULT Peel, trim, and quarter each cucumber. Cut into slices. Keep the slices from each cucumber separated.

CHILD Cut the slices of the first cucumber into a dice and repeat with the second cucumber, but keep them separated.

ADULT Place the herbs, garlic, onion, bell pepper, ½ cup (120 ml) of the water, and the slices from 1 of the cucumbers in the container of an electric stand blender, or place in a tall cylindrical container and use an immersion blender. Blend until well combined. Blend in the whole milk and season to taste with salt and pepper. Pour soup into a large bowl.

CHILD Add the remaining diced cucumber to the soup. Add 8 to 10 ice cubes and chill.

ADULT Serve in bowls, and garnish with edible flowers and fresh dill.

PREP TIME	YIELD
10 minutes	6 to 8 servings

{ DAY 11 } Become a Confident Cook

IF YOU DON'T LIKE TO COOK, you may lack confidence and skills, particularly some of the basic skills designed for ease and efficiency. If you are intimidated by cooking, you have two choices: Learn or be forever at the mercy of restaurants and packaged, prepared foods.

Like many chefs and great cooks, Lynn is not professionally trained; she learned by doing and watching others. As a food writer for magazines and newspapers, she interviewed and observed top chefs of many cuisines demonstrate their most famous recipes. Often, she collaborated with them to adapt recipes for the home cook.

Later, she took these chefs' secrets and shared them in our cooking education programs. For more than eighteen years, we have designed effective and popular cooking programs. We teach nutrition for all ages and guide families as they learn to cook together. Every recommendation we offer in this book has been tested successfully by thousands of families in our programs across the United States. Obviously we can't teach you everything you need to know about cooking in one chapter. So we're going to focus on the four areas that will help you the most: How to (1) read a recipe properly; (2) practice *mise en place* and organization; (3) measure properly; and (4) develop knife skills.

> **MISSION FOR THE DAY**
>
> Prepare a new recipe using an unfamiliar technique.

read and follow a recipe properly to get great results

Yes, there is a correct way to read a recipe. What could happen if you skip over this section? Quantities might be off, prep time might be prolonged, or something might burn because you were not aware that some items needed to be prepared in advance. Follow these steps to ensure great results:

- ♡ Before you start, read the recipe all the way through, from beginning to end.
- ♡ Understand that ingredients are listed in the order they are used.
- ♡ Follow the measurements; they are critical.
- ♡ After you have read the recipe, gather all the ingredients, pots, pans, bowls, and measuring utensils you will need.
- ♡ Double-check all the steps and ingredients.
- ♡ Follow the instructions and prep ingredients as required.

lynn's story

Time and again I hear mother's lament they don't have the time or energy to cook. I can relate. I, too, felt unable to cook meals after my divorce, even though I knew how to cook well. It seemed like too much work, and I had plenty of other responsibilities as a single parent. But I cooked because it was more economical, it provided real foods without additives, and homemade meals enhanced my family identity. Home cooking also developed my children's palates, shifting them away from the overly sugary and salty "kids' foods"— there was just "food."

Prepare Your *Mise En Place* to Save Time

Mise en place is a French term that means "to put in place." In culinary terms it means to have every ingredient out, washed, measured, and cut, and all your equipment and supplies ready as necessary. You should prepare your mise en place before you start a recipe. This gets your kids involved—they'll love to help you—and it saves time.

Measure Properly so Recipes Turn Out Right

Here are some important distinctions to help you understand the process of measuring:

- ♡ Dry ingredients are measured by weight. You'll need a set of nested (graduated) measuring cups in order to measure properly. In the United States these cups are made in the following sizes: ¼ cup, ⅓ cup, ½ cup, 1 cup, and 2 cups.
- ♡ Liquid ingredients are measured by volume. You'll need a clear glass or plastic cup with a pouring spout to measure liquids correctly. In the United States liquid measuring cups generally come in 1-, 2-, and 4- cup sizes.
- ♡ You'll need measuring spoons, too—your silverware isn't accurate enough. Measuring spoon

sizes in the United States include ⅛ teaspoon, ¼ teaspoon, ½ teaspoon, 1 teaspoon, and 1 tablespoon.

develop knife skills for time-saving efficiency

Learning knife skills will make all the difference and change your attitude about cooking with vegetables. Reluctant home cooks can transform into eager family chefs simply because they learned how to use a knife confidently!

Safety First

Learn how to handle knives safely by doing the following—injuries can definitely dampen your enthusiasm for cooking:

- ♡ **safe hand placement:** Always cut, chop, slice, or dice with the fingertips of your other hand curled down and in toward your palm, so that only the flat part of your knuckles face the blade.
- ♡ **keep knives sharp:** Sharp knives cut quickly, efficiently, and cleanly. They are safer. Dull knives can slip off the food and cause injury.
- ♡ **storage safety:** Store knives in a block or designated section of a drawer, never loose among other tools.

Rocking Motion

(See photos) This slicing technique uses a gentle rocking motion:

1. Hold the knife at a 45-degree angle. (A)
2. Come down swiftly through the food. (B)
3. Slide the knife down to the end of the blade near the handle.
4. Gently rock back along the blade to the knife tip.
5. Don't let the tip leave the cutting board.

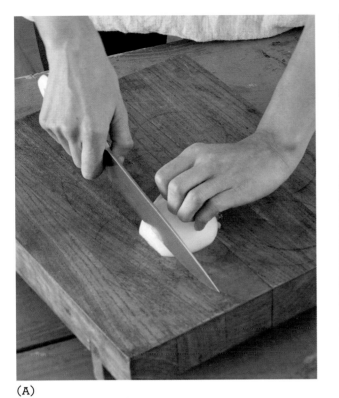

(A)

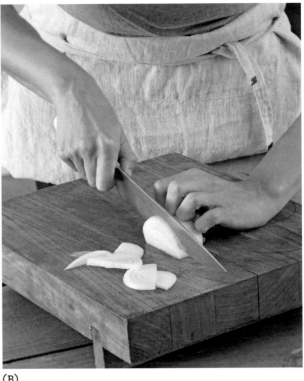

(B)

"This is my invariable advice to people: Learn how to cook—try new recipes, learn from your mistakes, be fearless, and above all have fun!" —Julia Child

Mincing

Many of the recipes in this book call for cutting veggies into very small pieces. Here's how to do it:

1. Holding your knife in one hand, balance four fingers of your other hand just under the knuckles on the tip end of the blade. (C)
2. Using the handle, rock the knife back and forth with your other hand acting as a stabilizer, keeping the tip down on the cutting board. (D)
3. As you rock, move the knife handle forward and back to mince the ingredients evenly.

Note: In addition to the photos here, you can watch many online videos that clearly present these basic techniques.

Developing true culinary skill and artistry takes focus, practice, and discipline. Keep these tips in mind, and you'll soon be on your way to preparing delicious and nutritious meals—and having fun in the process.

get started

Now that you've learned the basics, you're ready to put your new knowledge and skills to use:

- ♡ Make the salsa recipe in this chapter.
- ♡ Select a more advanced recipe such as risotto or Persian rice from Day 20 and prepare it with your children.
- ♡ Make a salad, main course, and dessert from scratch, including a simple fruit dessert from the recipes in Day 19.

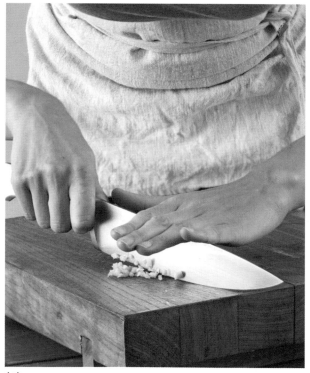

(C)

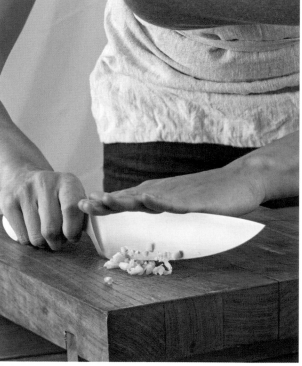

(D)

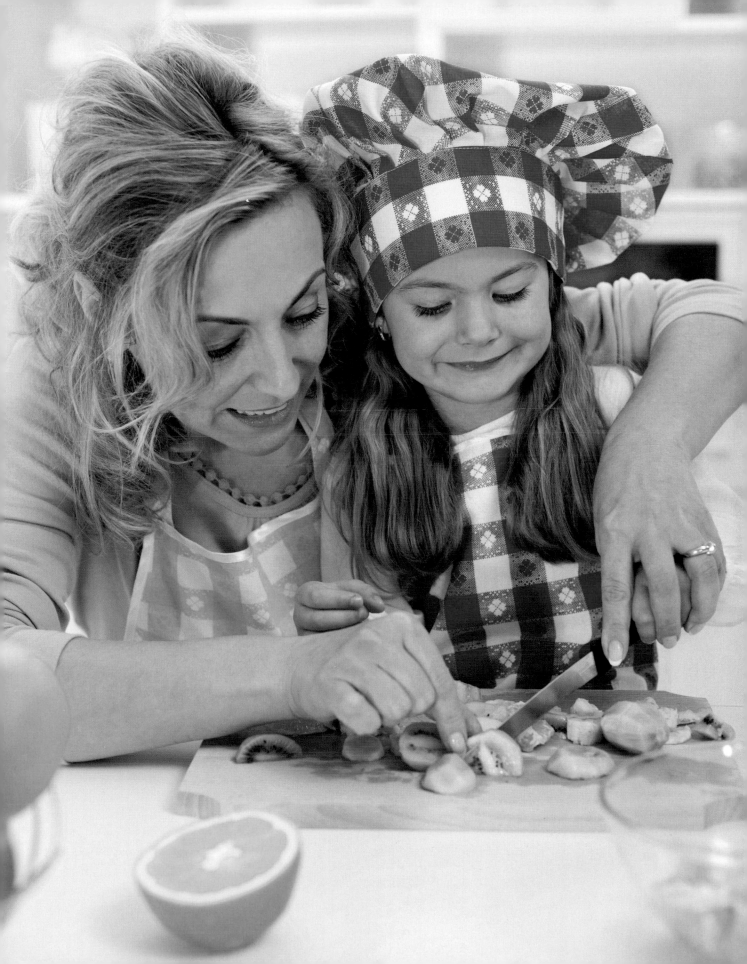

persian new year soup

In the Persian culture, this recipe is prepared as part of the ritual of welcoming spring at the equinox, marking the earth's passage out of winter. You will have some extra legumes and root veggies, so add them to one of our salad concepts.

1 medium onion

1 tablespoon (15 ml) olive oil

4 cups (946 ml) beef or vegetable broth

¼ teaspoon turmeric

½ cup (128 g) canned kidney beans

½ cup (128 g) canned white beans

½ cup (120 g) canned chickpeas

¼ cup (48 g) dried lentils, soaked for a couple hours

Kosher salt and freshly ground black pepper

4 scallions

1 bunch fresh dill

1 bunch fresh parsley

⅔ cup (60 g) thawed and drained frozen spinach, or ½ pound (225 g) fresh, cleaned, cooked, and drained

½ beet

¼ pound (115 g) Reshteh (Persian noodles) or linguine

2 tablespoons (12 g) flour

2 tablespoons (30 ml) vinegar, or to taste

NOTE: *Children should use plastic or table knives for all child steps that require cutting or chopping.*

ADULT Slice the onion into thin strips.

ADULT Heat the olive oil in a large saucepan over medium heat.

ADULT & CHILD Add the onion and cook, stirring frequently, about 10 to 15 minutes, or until golden brown.

ADULT & CHILD Add the broth, turmeric, kidney beans, white beans, chickpeas, and lentils; salt and pepper to taste. Cook for 10 minutes.

CHILD While the beans are cooking, slice the scallions or snip them with scissors.

CHILD Chop the dill, parsley, and spinach (if you are using fresh).

CHILD Dice the beet.

ADULT & CHILD Add dill, parsley, spinach, and beet to the pot, and take turns stirring the soup.

ADULT Season to taste with salt and pepper as the mixture cooks.

ADULT & CHILD Add the noodles and flour. Cook for about 7 more minutes, or until noodles are done.

CHILD Stir in vinegar to taste.

ADULT To serve, ladle into bowls.

PREP TIME	COOK TIME	YIELD
27 minutes	20 minutes	4 servings

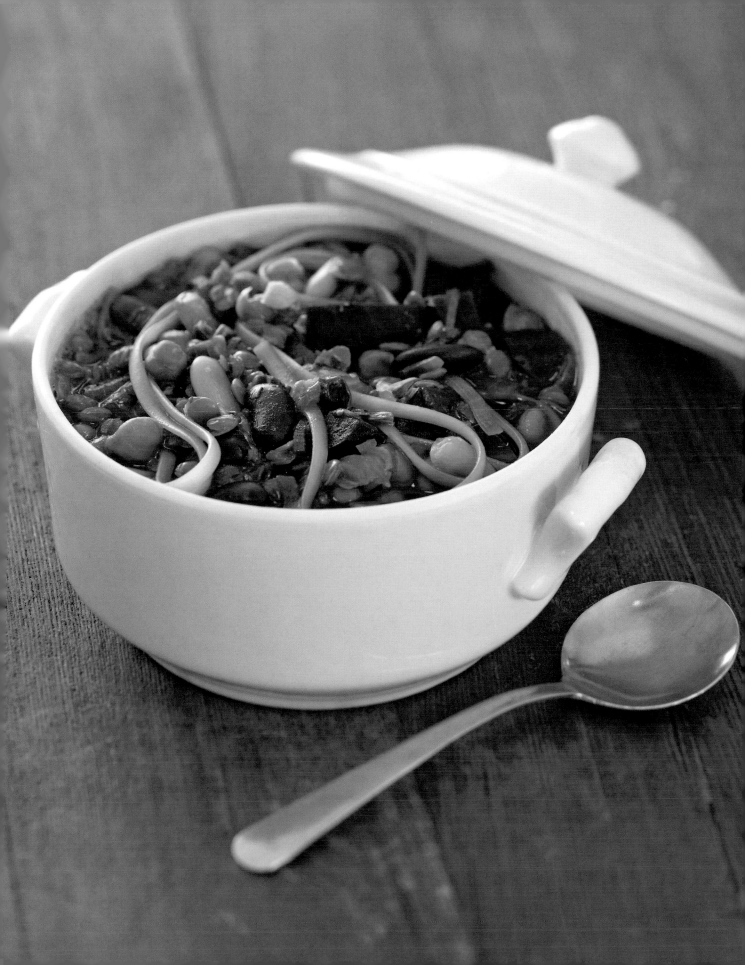

caribbean salsa and steamed snapper

Children love this recipe because it is colorful and so much fun to make. Serve the salsa with tortilla chips for a snack—it's more than an accompaniment for fish.

FOR SALSA:

1 can (14 ounces, or 397 g) black beans

1 can (14 ounces, or 397 g) corn

1 ripe mango

1 medium red onion

2 plum tomatoes

1 red bell pepper

1 bunch cilantro

4 limes

6 tablespoons (90 ml) pineapple juice

Kosher salt

FOR SNAPPER:

1 tablespoon (15 ml) vegetable oil

3 snapper fillets, 8 ounces (225 g) each

Kosher salt and freshly ground pepper

ADDITIONAL COOKING EQUIPMENT:
Bamboo or metal steamer

NOTE: *Children should use plastic or table knives for all child steps that require cutting or chopping.*

TO MAKE THE SALSA:

ADULT Strain the beans and corn in a colander and rinse well, then place in a large mixing bowl.

ADULT Peel the mango and onion.

ADULT Slice the onion, tomatoes, red pepper, and mango.

ADULT & CHILD Dice the onion, tomatoes, bell pepper, and mango and add to the mixing bowl.

CHILD Pluck the cilantro leaves from their stems and add to the bowl.

CHILD Squeeze limes into a measuring cup to yield ⅓ cup (80 ml) lime juice. Add to the salsa.

CHILD Add the pineapple juice to the salsa, adjusting amount to taste, and stir with a wooden spoon.

ADULT & CHILD Season with salt to taste.

TO MAKE THE STEAMED SNAPPER:

ADULT & CHILD Help prepare the bamboo steamer and oil each chamber's bottom surface so the fish will not stick. If using a metal steamer, oil it on the side where you will lay the fish.

ADULT Heat about an inch (2.5 cm) of water in a pot large enough to fit the steamer. The water must be simmering before you add the fish.

ADULT Season the fillets with salt and pepper. Using a long-handled spatula, place the fillets skin side down into the bamboo steamer chambers or metal steamer.

CHILD Cover the steamer and cook about 5 to 7 minutes, or until flesh is opaque and flaky.

ADULT Open the steamer with an oven mitt and tongs.

ADULT Serve immediately with Caribbean Salsa. Some children may not want the salsa on the fish; it can be served either on top or on the side.

PREP TIME	COOK TIME	YIELD
20 minutes	5 to 7 minutes	15 small servings

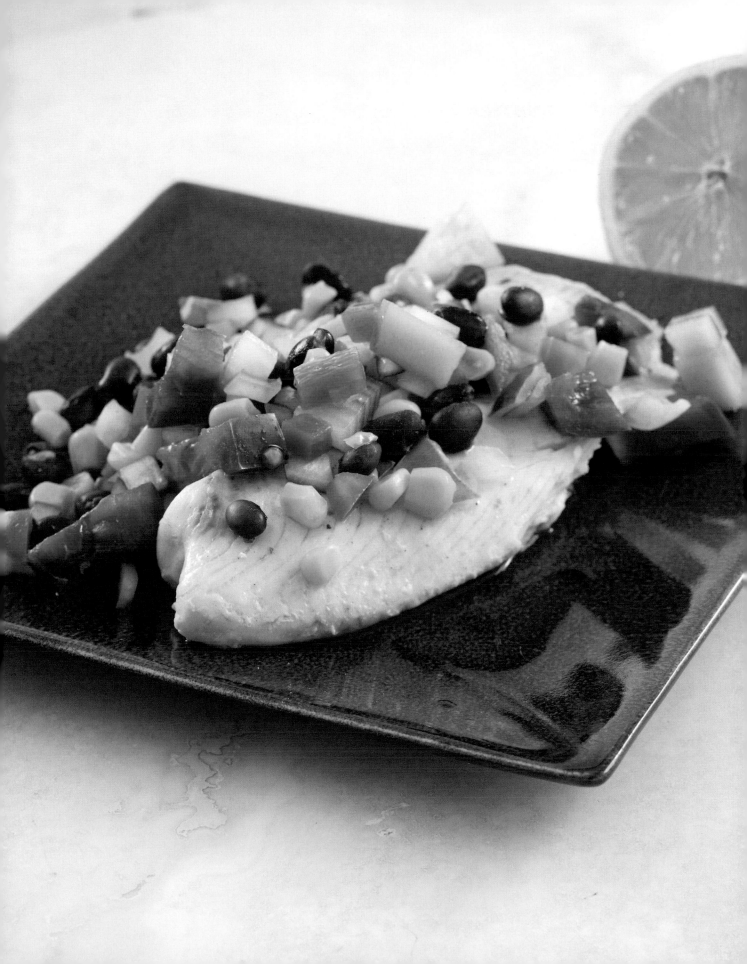

chocolate chip carrot cake

Lynn's best friend from college, Linda Levy, introduced her to this fantastic recipe years ago, and it's always a hit at parties.

2 large bunches carrots

1⅓ cups (315 ml) canola oil

2 cups (400 g) sugar

4 eggs

3 cups (298 g) flour

2½ teaspoons (6 g) ground cinnamon

4 teaspoons (18 g) baking powder

1 teaspoon baking soda

1 package (12 ounces, or 340 g) semisweet chocolate chips

1 tablespoon (14 g) butter

ADDITIONAL COOKING EQUIPMENT:
1 large tube pan; box grater or food processor

NOTE: *Children should use plastic or table knives for all child steps that require cutting or chopping.*

ADULT Preheat oven to 350°F (180°C, or gas mark 4).

ADULT & CHILD Peel and grate the carrots with a box grater or in a food processor. If using a grater, let young children help by holding the end of the veggies while you hold their hands and help them go up and down once or twice. Older children can do this independently.

CHILD Help measure the oil and sugar into a large mixing bowl. Mix well and then add the grated carrots. Mix thoroughly.

ADULT & CHILD Crack the eggs on edge of a bowl; with two thumbs in the crack, the child can separate the halves and drop the eggs into the bowl. Add to the carrot mixture and mix well.

CHILD Help measure the flour, cinnamon, baking powder, and baking soda into a separate large mixing bowl.

ADULT & CHILD Mix the dry ingredients well. Add to the carrot mixture, 1 cup at a time, mixing thoroughly between additions until all is well blended.

CHILD Add the chocolate chips. Mix well.

ADULT & CHILD Grease a large tube pan with the butter. Pour in the batter.

ADULT Bake in preheated oven for 60 to 90 minutes, or until a toothpick inserted into the center comes out dry.

PREP TIME	COOK TIME	YIELD
20 minutes	1 to 1 ½ hours	About 15 servings

{DAY 12} Empower Your Sous Chefs

Cooking and tasting engages all the senses and encourages eating new foods

One of the biggest dividends of letting children cook is a shift from being wary of new foods to being open to eating them. The acceptance of a particular food starts during the stage of hands-on cooking experience, by touching, smelling, and tasting the food before it is cooked. Cutting, squeezing and using herbs, spices, and fresh ingredients enhances the fragrances and encourages children to taste. Tangible, multi-sensory experiences make learning come alive for children. Our FamilyCook programs employ all that Lynn learned from her own kitchen laboratory and from cooking with hundreds of families. Our school-based classes for children are not demos. Each child participates in every aspect of making each recipe. They measure ingredients, grate carrots and sliver cucumbers into matchsticks. You and your children can become a happy team trying out new recipes because they offer new ways to manipulate foods, new smells and tastes, and new, cool cooking tools.

Cooking together saves time

It is not as unusual to bring kids into the kitchen today as it was when Lynn started twenty years ago. But for many families, such activities are reserved for baking or for holidays when there is more time. However, after some practice, you'll see you actually shave off valuable minutes in meal preparation

MISSION FOR THE DAY

Invite your children to help you cook a meal or snack.

thanks to the extra support from your sous chefs! Being offered a real 'job' makes children proud to make a contribution to the family meal and hence excited to do their best and show parents that they can be trusted to participate.

You'll make another important discovery, too. Children learn through repetition, so they love to execute the more repetitive tasks that adults often find boring and tedious. No more lettuce washing

lynn's story

I discovered the transformative effects of family cooking quite by accident after my divorce; when my younger son, Stephan, was a toddler and my older son, Alex, was seven. I longed for a way to connect with my boys, and enjoy being a family, beyond the daily routines of dressing, bathing, and reminding them to pick up their socks.

Sadly, in the initial months after the split, I too often served dinner to television-entranced children and retreated to my room or called my mother to vent. This was not how I had envisioned parenthood. Nor did it resemble how I had been raised. (continued on page 92)

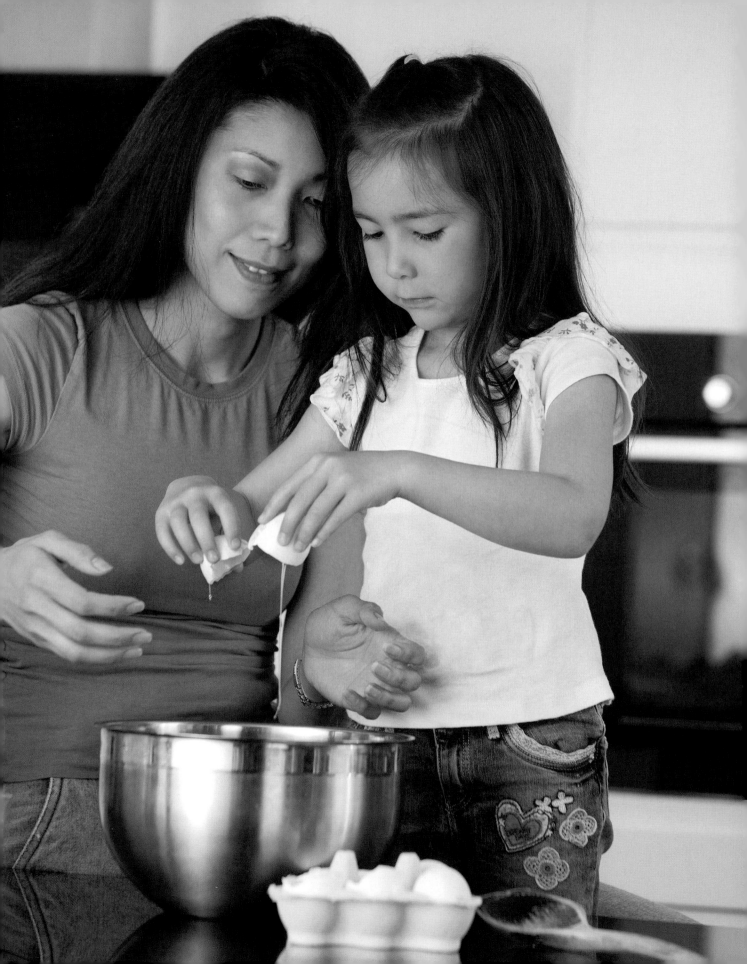

cooking tasks for children of all ages

tasks	toddler, preschool age (2 to 5 years)	school age (6 to 10 years)	adolescent (11 to 17 years)
prepare herbs, lettuce, and other greens	Snip herbs; tear up leaves separated from the head	Snip herbs; wash, dry, separate, and tear the leaves	Snip herbs; wash, dry, separate, and tear the leaves
prepare raw vegetables	Snap green beans in half; help cut up thinly sliced vegetables using table knife	Snap ends off green beans and cut in half with table knife; cut up sliced vegetables with table knife	Snap off the ends of green beans and slice in half with paring knife; slice or dice vegetables with knives, with supervision
measure	Hold cups and spoons while adult pours	Help measure dry ingredients	Measure liquid and dry ingredients
stir in a bowl or pot	Take turns counting 1, 2, 3	Take alternating turns with adult	Perform task independently
grate vegetables or cheese with box grater	Take turns counting 1, 2, 3	Take alternating turns with adult	Perform task independently
use a blender or food processor	Push a button	Push buttons sequentially	Operate the blender independently
use an electric hand mixer	Help parent hold the mixer	Take alternating turns holding mixer with adult	Operate hand mixer with minimum supervision
use a manual chopper	Help parent push down	Take alternating turns with adult	Operate independently
use a pasta machine	Help adult turn the crank	Turn the crank with supervision	Operate with supervision
juice citrus by hand or machine	Help squeeze citrus	Squeeze fruit until tired	Perform task independently
cut meat	N/A	Help cut up a piece or two with table knife	Cut up pieces of meat using knives, with supervision
clean shrimp or mussels	Squeeze mussel shells to make sure mussels are alive	Help pull off shells and help devein shrimp	Shell and devein shrimp; remove mussels from shells independently

The pivotal incident seemed, at the time, an act of desperation. Yet it was so simple: I handed twenty-month-old Stephan a bunch of basil and told him he could "help" me cook. He'd been restlessly playing with pots on the floor and was thrilled to sit at the table and pluck the leaves off the stems.

After ten minutes of observing his contentment-which gave me the freedom to cook without being pressured by a whining toddler—I was sold. In the ensuing days and weeks, I tried out numerous cooking tasks that could be safely adapted for a toddler, tasks that also provided a sense of accomplishment for Stephan so he felt part of the process.

After I'd established his role in the kitchen, I sought a way to entice my older son to join us. Asking him to help his little brother wasn't going to work, so I took Alex food shopping. I let him choose the family's meals for the next three days. He felt so empowered! His choices included some foods that were routine for the family, plus a few new items. I grew excited as I saw a way for my new family of three to get out of our rut. Now the notion of cooking time being family time was at last coming full circle and we never looked back.

doing homework, or hanging out. Lynn explained to her boys that at dinner time the kitchen is where she could be found. Before long they got into the rhythm of turning the television off at dinnertime and joining her in the kitchen to cook, do some homework, and have her complete attention. This last was the number one draw, they all connected as a family more deeply during this time of day and were contented.

age-appropriate tasks get everyone involved

To make sure everyone gets a chance to participate and experience the pride of accomplishment, choose age-appropriate tasks that kids can handle. Young children require lots of supervision, but as they age they gain more confidence and independence. By the time they reach their teens, many are quite capable of making entire meals by themselves. The easy-reference chart on page 91 shows appropriate cooking tasks for children of different ages.

get started
Select a recipe in this book that you think everyone will enjoy preparing together. Here are some ways to involve your children:

♡ Think about the tasks you find most tedious—which can you delegate to kids? Review the directions for child steps.
♡ Share the job of cooking with your children—they will be excited and proud to be included.

and chopping veggies--your children will be thrilled to do that for you! They will also peel all your carrots, tear all your greens, and grate your cheese. Sure it will take some practice, but you will be shocked just how short their learning curve can be. The incentive, apart from spending time with you, isthe allure of fresh fish topped with colorful salsa they chopped themselves.

It is also important to let kids know they are not expected to cook with you especially once the initial novelty of cooking wears off. Rather, kids should feel there is an open invitation to help and just be in the kitchen with you whether they are cooking,

fruit kebabs

Very young children will enjoy helping cut the fruit and thread it onto coffee stirrers, which make safe skewers. Try some preschool math with them: ask them to create different patterns by repeating and alternating fruit of various colors and shapes on the skewers. You can vary this recipe by using fruits your children prefer.

1 orange

1 banana

1 small bunch red grapes

SPECIAL EQUIPMENT:
Plastic coffee stirrers (about 1 dozen)

NOTE: *Children should use plastic or table knives for all child steps that require cutting or chopping.*

ADULT & CHILD Peel the orange and banana. Break orange into sections, and cut the banana into 1-inch (2.5 cm) pieces.

CHILD Help cut the orange segments in half. Place in a mixing bowl.

CHILD Help cut the banana into smaller, bite-size pieces. Add to the same bowl.

CHILD Help cut the grapes in half. Add to the bowl.

CHILD Choose a piece of fruit and push it onto a coffee stirrer. Add different fruits, alternating in a pleasing pattern (about 6 pieces per stirrer, depending on size of fruit).

CHILD Continue until all the fruit is used. Enjoy for a snack with family and friends.

PREP TIME	YIELD
10 minutes	8 to 12 kebabs

meatless bolognese with penne

The tofu in this recipe soaks up the sweetness of the carrots and creates a wonderful, hearty, textured sauce that is a huge success with all ages.

1 onion

3 carrots

2 tablespoons (30 ml) extra-virgin olive oil

1 jar (26 ounces, or 765 ml) marinara sauce

1 package (8 ounces, or 225 g) firm tofu

⅓ cup (80 ml) milk, or to taste

Nutmeg, freshly grated (or pregrated)

Kosher salt

¾ pound (340 g) penne pasta, cooked and drained

NOTE: *Children should use plastic or table knives for all child steps that require cutting or chopping.*

ADULT Slice the onion.

CHILD Help chop the onion.

CHILD Help grate the carrots.

ADULT Heat the olive oil in a medium saucepan over low heat. Add onions and cook 5 minutes. Add grated carrots and cook 5 minutes more.

ADULT & CHILD Add the marinara sauce to the saucepan. Stir carefully, using a long-handled wooden spoon and wearing oven mitts. Turn heat up to medium and cook for 5 minutes.

ADULT & CHILD Crumble the tofu into the sauce. Mix thoroughly. Cook over medium heat another 5 to 7 minutes, or until sauce begins to simmer.

ADULT & CHILD Measure and pour the milk into the sauce, adding more to taste.

ADULT & CHILD Grate the nutmeg and stir into sauce. Season to taste with salt. Serve over penne pasta.

tips

• You can make this recipe in advance as it keeps well refrigerated or frozen.

• Look for jar sauce that does not have added sugar.

PREP TIME	COOK TIME	YIELD
15 minutes	25 minutes	6 to 8 servings

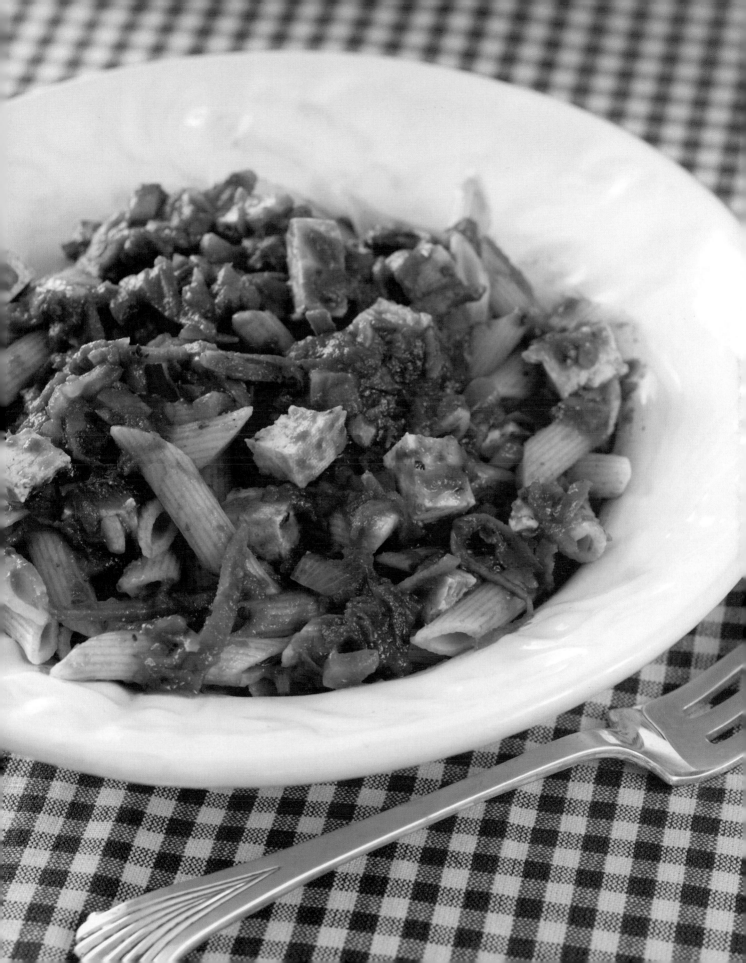

PART 4

FOCUS ON WHOLE FOODS FOR HEALTHIER MEALS

{DAY 13} Add More Veggies to Your Family's Diet

LEFT TO THEIR OWN DEVICES, our children might only want to eat what they see advertised on TV or what's in those brightly colored packages on the supermarket shelves. But by now you've learned ways to encourage your children to try new and healthier foods, especially fruits and vegetables. Taking family field trips to the farmers' market and inviting your kids to help you cook and plan meals can make them more open to experimentation. Such intentional strategies engage all their senses and familiarize kids with real, whole foods that will keep their bodies healthy.

You can also adopt some of the tactics marketing pros use to attract youngsters. The chart on page 98 offers suggestions for using food marketers' strategies to shift your kids away from junk food and over to fruits and veggies.

Introducing new varieties and greater quantities of vegetables to children's diets can be particularly challenging. Luckily, we can learn from other cultures. In other parts of the world, where the food culture is entwined with national pride and family traditions, food marketers have a harder time breaking in. Fast foods and junk foods are there, but they have less impact.

MISSION FOR THE DAY

Entice your children to eat a new vegetable.

mercedes' story

I grew up in Spain, and I associate stews, omelets, cocido (chickpeas), and other foods with the pleasure my relatives experienced while preparing and eating these foods. These dishes are served in school, at friends' homes, and in restaurants across Spain. As I child I was not wild about some of the vegetables. But as I grew up, I started to eat them because they were familiar and I associated them with family enjoyment.

Today, when my American children vacation in Spain, they associate paella, gazpacho, melons, and other typical Spanish foods with our summers there. They thrill with the pleasure of eating these foods with the extended family. Food marketers in the United States bombard children with ads that feature celebrities or superheroes, but the Spanish culture bombards its young people with its wealth of national dishes. The key difference is authenticity—my aunt and siblings are not paid to swoon over the paellas they create! For my kids, given the choice of paella or a fast-food hamburger, paella would win every time.

become a "master marketer" of healthy food to your family

marketers' strategies	use their strategies to get kids to eat healthy
familiarity ads and junk food logos displayed everywhere—phones, facebook, school, tv, movies, computer games	Frequently serve and provide the healthy foods you want your children to eat. These foods should always be in your cupboards and refrigerator. Turn on the Food Channel and watch programs that show chefs cooking real food. Plant a vegetable garden so veggies are familiar and exciting.
accessibility junk food sold everywhere you go, from your corner store to a mountain resort, especially at the supermarket checkout aisle	Wherever you go and however you travel with your children (to the park, in the car, in the subway, on a plane or bus), bring your own delicious food to keep them from begging for junk food. We don't buy food on the highway; we always bring sandwiches, fruits, crudités, and drinks.
reachable junk food displayed at eye level and easy for kids to reach in the store	Keep veggies cut up and within reach. Keep a bowl of fruit, cherry tomatoes, or snap peas in the kitchen and living room at all times. Fresh food should always be available when children are hungry.

In Europe, for instance, people as a whole aren't likely to choose highly processed foods for meals. Packaged snacks have become more popular, but at mealtime Europeans usually make regional dishes—mostly prepared with whole foods—that are linked to their national identity. From Scandinavia to Greece, traditional home-cooked recipes play a significant role at holidays, rituals, and celebrations. Familiar, accessible foods plus the pleasurable experience of eating together as a family encourage children to enjoy national recipes—many of them loaded with vegetables.

try international one-pot dishes that make veggies appealing

American culture tends to emphasize meat- or cheese-based meals; vegetables rarely make up the main dish, except in some soups and casseroles. Rather, vegetables are served on the side, unceremoniously. Yet the United States has a multiplicity of cultures and traditions, and each has its own creative and delectable recipes that incorporate vegetables with grains and meats.

Our recipe concepts offer festive meals that introduce new veggies that may not be familiar to you. Experiment with them and find your family favorites. Once your kids get used to eating one-pot meals that combine everything, they'll get tired of picking out what they don't like and become resigned to the idea that this is how they're going to eat.

Wouldn't it be amazing to see your children enthusiastic about eating their veggies? As Mercedes explained earlier, in Spain people tend to eat foods that are familiar, accessible, and associated with pleasurable experiences. Food marketers have used the same ideas—familiarity, accessibility, and pleasure—with great success.

In our classes, we evoke pleasurable memories, using a multicultural approach. Nutrition is presented in a positive and celebratory way as an intrinsic part of each culture's diet. You can do the same thing at home by introducing exotic, colorful, and uniquely shaped vegetables to your children in a celebratory way.

spicy kenyan greens

We adapted this recipe from several Kenyan recipes, using greens with a hint of spice. The fresh jalapeño adds a delightful zing to the dish.

1 jalapeño pepper

2 teaspoons (12 g) salt

2 teaspoons (4 g) freshly ground black pepper

2 tablespoons (30 ml) extra-virgin olive oil, divided

1 pound (454 g) leafy greens (kale, collards, mustard, chard)

1 pound (455 g) spinach

3 large tomatoes

1 large yellow onion

2 tablespoons (28 g) butter

1 can (13 to 15 ounces, or 369 to 430 g) coconut milk

Salt and freshly ground black pepper

4 teaspoons (14 g) chopped dry roasted peanuts (optional)

NOTE: *Children should use plastic or table knives for all child steps that require cutting or chopping.*

ADULT Chop the jalapeño (protect hands with plastic gloves) and discard seeds. Measure 1 cup (235 ml) water into a large skillet or wok. Add the jalapeño.

CHILD Help measure salt, black pepper, and 1 tablespoon (15 ml) of the olive oil. Add to pan with the water and jalapeño.

ADULT Bring the water to boil over high heat.

ADULT & CHILD Chop or tear all the greens, including the spinach. Add to the pot.

ADULT Cook the greens for 3 minutes, or until they begin to wilt. Drain and cool.

ADULT While the greens are cooking, slice the tomatoes and onion.

ADULT & CHILD Dice the sliced tomatoes and onion.

ADULT Heat the remaining 1 tablespoon (15 ml) of olive oil and the butter in separate very large skillet over medium heat. Add the cooled greens and spinach, chopped tomatoes, onions, and coconut milk; stir together. Cook 3 to 5 minutes, until flavors meld. Season to taste with salt and pepper.

ADULT Serve with a sprinkle of chopped peanuts on each serving.

PREP TIME	COOK TIME	YIELD
15 minutes	20 minutes	6 to 8 servings

spicy corn salad

Hot peppers give this colorful salad a spicy Southwestern flavor that complements the smoked fish.

2 leeks, or 1 onion

2 tablespoons (30 ml) extra-virgin olive oil

2 cloves garlic

3 ears sweet corn

1 jalapeño, or ½ habañero, or Scotch bonnet, pepper

1 red, orange, or yellow bell pepper

1 yellow squash

1 large tomato

½ cup (16 g) cilantro

1 can (4 to 5 ounces, or 115 to 140 g) smoked trout, or 4 ounces (115 g) smoked salmon

Kosher salt

¼ teaspoon freshly ground black pepper

NOTE: *Children should use plastic or table knives for all child steps that require cutting or chopping.*

ADULT Clean and slice the leeks thinly, or chop the onion.

ADULT Heat a large skillet over medium-low heat and add the olive oil.

ADULT Add the leeks and cook slowly. Smash and slice the garlic with the flat side of a chef's knife to remove the peel; slice the garlic.

ADULT & CHILD Finely chop the garlic slices. Add to pan.

ADULT Slice the bottoms of the corn off the cobs and stand each on the flat bottom. Slice the kernels off the ears of corn and add them to pan. Cook and stir until softened.

ADULT Slice the jalapeño (wear protective gloves). Add to the pan. If using habañero, discard the seeds.

ADULT Slice the bell pepper, squash, and tomato into thin slices.

CHILD Cut the bell pepper slices into a small dice. Stack the squash slices and slice into strips, turn, and slice into a small dice. Repeat this step with the tomatoes.

ADULT Add vegetables to the pan, and cook and stir for 3 minutes.

CHILD Pluck the cilantro leaves from the stems. Chop the leaves and add them to the pan.

CHILD Help flake the smoked fish or salmon and add it to the pot.

ADULT & CHILD Turn off the heat, and season to taste with salt and pepper.

PREP TIME	COOK TIME	YIELD
20 minutes	10 minutes	10 servings

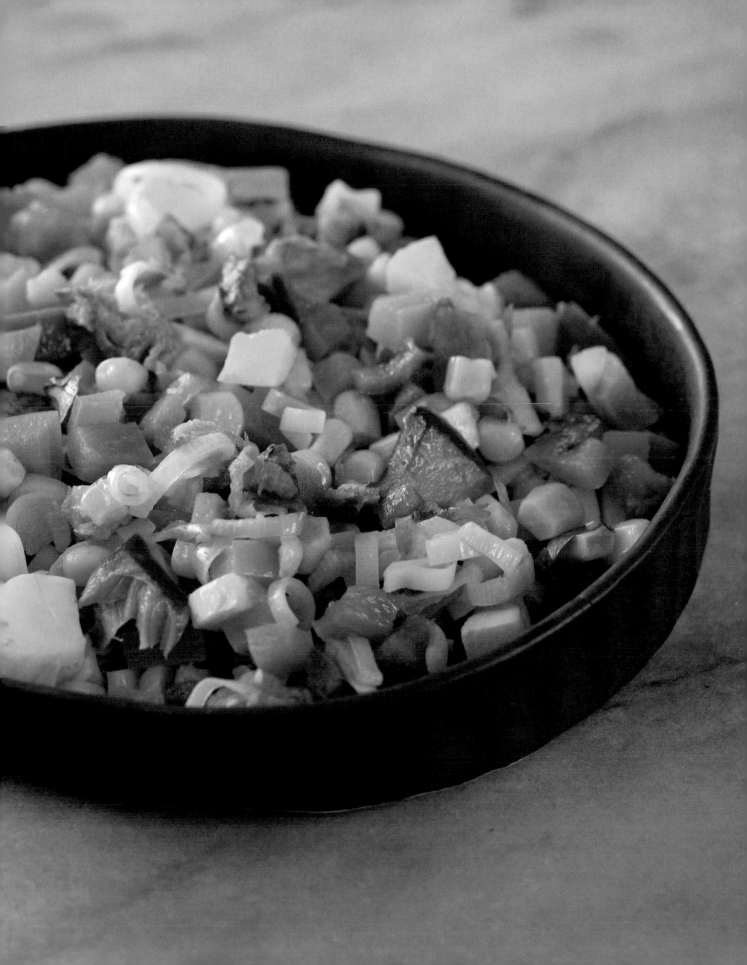

{ DAY 14 } Soup Up for Tasty Nutrition

HOMEMADE SOUPS are some of the easiest and healthiest meals you can prepare—and many types can be made quickly and easily. Soups provide balanced nutrition and give you an opportunity to sneak new veggies and flavors into your family's diet. Soup is a comfort food, and usually nonthreatening to children. Lynn considers soup her secret weapon. She discovered she could pack it with all the veggies she wanted, and so long as it tasted delicious, her boys would gobble it down.

If your children don't like one particular veggie, purée-style soups are the answer. When you blend everything into one nutritious elixir, that disliked vegetable's taste is masked, and it's impossible for your kids to remove anything. A chunky-style soup presents a different challenge to picky eaters. For the most part, picking out the offending veggie—be it kale, beans, or onions—is pretty annoying and time consuming. When Lynn suggested that her sons just "eat around it," they generally complied. The nutrients remained in the broth, despite the pains they took to avoid eating what they didn't like.

Soup is a great way to use up leftovers, either as an ingredient or on the side. You can serve soup for dinner to supplement leftover meat from a roast, or serve roasted chicken or turkey on the side. Soups are some of the most successful and popular recipes in this book, both with our own children and with families nationwide. These recipes are very colorful, celebratory, culturally focused, and include a wide variety of ingredients.

soup offers a quick solution to mealtime dilemmas Once you've developed your repertoire and confidence, you can make a soup on the fly and reduce mealtime stress. Simply see what's in your fridge and decide which version to make—chunky or puréed—and you can check off "dinner" from your to-do list.

In truth we've been brainwashed by the convenience of canned, cubed, powdered, and prepared versions. But before these so-called conveniences, people simply combined vegetables, legumes, and meats with water, added their favorite herbs, spices, or other flavorings to the pot, put the lid on, and left the rest to the magic of heat and time.

You can make simple purée-style soups anytime, even when you are in a hurry.

🕐 get started

Get everyone involved in creating original soup recipes that will become family favorites:

- ♡ Select a basic recipe from pages 103 or 104
- ♡ Make a batch and divide it in half and create two different versions for your family to try.
- ♡ Consider buying an immersion blender. You will save time and effort.

potato leek soup purée

This basic recipe is tasty as is, but challenge yourself and your family to come up with varieties on this theme that will keep things interesting. (See box.)

2 leeks

2 tablespoons (28 g) butter

1 tablespoon (15 ml) extra-virgin olive oil

3 to 4 medium russet potatoes

3 to 4 cups (705 to 946 ml) water, chicken or vegetable broth, or other liquid

Salt and freshly ground pepper

ADDITIONAL COOKING EQUIPMENT: Immersion or electric blender, or food processor

NOTE: *Children should use plastic or table knives for all child steps that require cutting or chopping.*

ADULT Slice leeks thinly. Heat the butter and oil in a large saucepan over high heat. Add the leeks, reduce heat to low, and cook about 10 minutes, or until leeks are softened.

CHILD Meanwhile, peel the potatoes.

ADULT & CHILD Adult slices the potatoes and child cuts slices in half.

ADULT Add the potatoes to the softened leeks and cook together for 5 minutes. Add the desired liquid. Bring to a boil then reduce heat. Simmer about 15 minutes, or until potatoes are very tender.

ADULT Purée in the pot with an immersion blender, or transfer to the container of a food processor or blender and purée in batches. Add additional liquid to thin until desired consistency is reached.

ADULT Reheat over medium heat until just bubbly. Season to taste with salt and pepper.

ADULT To serve, ladle into individual soup bowls. Add desired garnish.

variations

- Potato leek soup with balsamic vinegar: Make the base recipe and add a swirl of crème fraîche or heavy cream to each serving. Drizzle on a quality thick-style balsamic vinegar or glaze.

- Potato leek soup with cilantro or basil oil: Prepare the base recipe and add a swirl of crème fraîche or heavy cream. Using an electric blender or an immersion blender in a tall cylindrical container, blend together ¼ cup (60 ml) water, 10 large basil leaves or ⅓ cup (5 g) cilantro leaves, ¼ cup (60 ml) extra-virgin olive oil, and ½ teaspoon salt. Blend until liquid and pourable. Drizzle onto each serving.

- Potato leek soup with anise beet: Prepare the base recipe and add a swirl of crème fraîche or heavy cream. Using an electric blender or an immersion blender in a tall cylindrical container, blend together ¼ cup (60 ml) water, 1 small boiled beet, ½ teaspoon of anise seed, and ½ tablespoon extra-virgin olive oil. Blend until liquid and pourable, adding more water as needed. Drizzle over each serving, and garnish with a sprig of dill, chervil, or mint.

PREP TIME	COOK TIME	YIELD
15 minutes	30 minutes	4 to 6 servings

squash soup purée

The inherent sweetness of winter squash is appealing to children. Once they've helped to prepare this recipe, they'll want to taste their delicious creation.

1 medium onion

3 tablespoons (45 ml) olive oil

1 to 2 pounds (455 to 907 g) butternut squash

3 cups (710 ml) water, chicken or vegetable broth, or other liquid

Salt

1 tablespoon (14 g) butter

ADDITIONAL COOKING EQUIPMENT: Immersion or electric blender, or food processor

NOTE: *Children should use plastic or table knives for all child steps that require cutting or chopping.*

ADULT Slice the onion very thinly.

CHILD Chop the sliced onion into small dice.

ADULT Heat the olive oil in a medium saucepan over high heat. Add the onions, reduce heat to low, and cook about 10 minutes, or until translucent and browned.

ADULT & CHILD Meanwhile, peel the butternut squash. Remove seeds with a spoon (reserve and toast). Clean away the membrane, and slice into half circle rings. Cut the rings into cubes.

ADULT When the onions are cooked, add the liquid and the squash; season to taste with salt. Bring to a boil, reduce heat to low, and simmer about 4 to 7 minutes, or until squash is very tender.

ADULT Purée with immersion blender, or transfer to the container of a food processor or blender and purée in batches. Add additional liquid to thin until desired consistency is reached. Tranfer back into the saucepan and heat until just bubbly.

CHILD Measure and add the butter; stir until melted.

ADULT Serve in individual soup bowls with desired garnish.

variations

- Butternut squash and cider soup with feta: Peel and chop an apple, add to the onions, and sauté until soft. Continue to prepare as in the base recipe, using apple cider for liquid. Top each with feta and dill.

- Butternut squash soup with garam masala: Prepare as in the base recipe, but add 4 cups (.95 L) chicken broth as liquid. Before serving, add 2 teaspoons garam masala (Indian spice blend), and season to taste with salt and pepper. Add a swirl of crème fraîche to each serving.

- Chipotle butternut squash soup: Slice and chop 2 ribs celery, 1 carrot, and 2 cloves of garlic. Sauté with the onion in olive oil until very soft. Add squash and desired liquid and cook as in the base recipe. Season with 2 teaspoons chipotle chili powder. Finish with a swirl of Greek yogurt. Then garnish with toasted pumpkin seeds in each bowl.

PREP TIME	COOK TIME	YIELD
15 minutes	25 minutes	4 to 6 servings

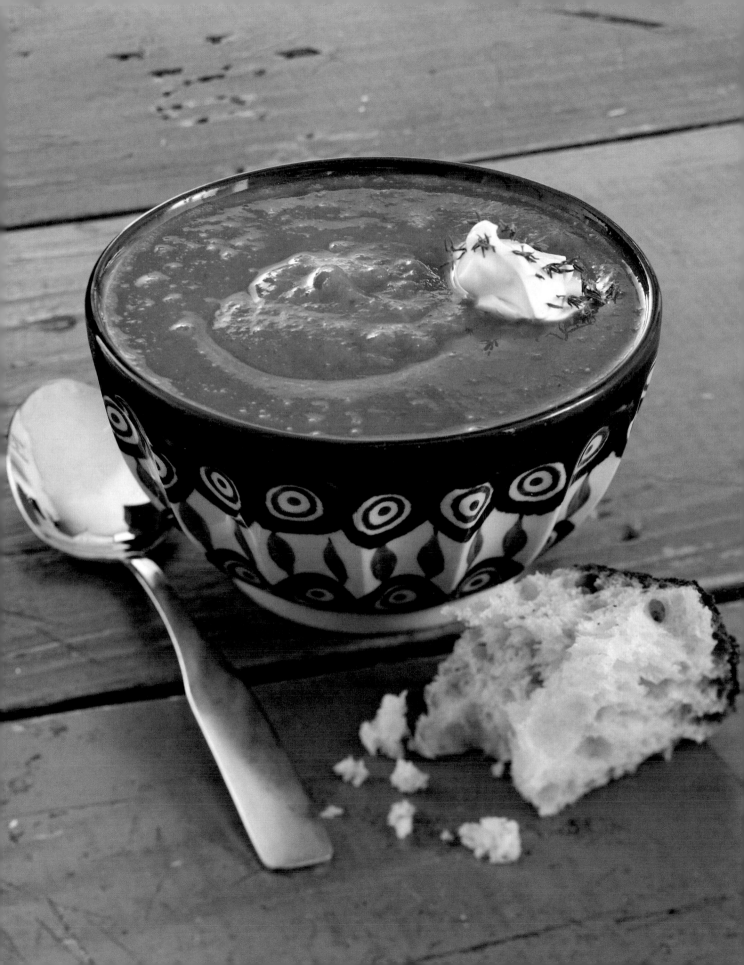

Master Your Salad Repertoire

OUR SALADS don't look like the lettuce-tomato-cucumber concoctions most people eat. Instead, ours are chock full of our favorite vegetables or created to showcase one or more specific vegetables or greens. Beets, kale, tender corn niblets, herbs, smoked fish, grilled chicken—you name the ingredient, and it will find its way into our salads.

Our "concept" approach has been highly successful in our educational programs. Parents of preschoolers in our "1, 2, 3, Nibble with Willow" program are amazed that their young, veggie-averse children will *ask* for more kale salad. Teens, after hands-on preparation, are amazed to discover they actually like a huge variety of new foods, and they love to share this new-found veggie love by cooking demonstrations at farmers' markets.

salad concepts make meal planning quick and exciting

We include five basic salad concepts in this chapter: composed salads, chopped salads, tomato salads, cruciferous salads, and bread salads. The beauty of our concepts is that you can change them, using whatever ingredients are in season, to keep your salads interesting throughout the year.

Composed Salads Are Fun to Fix

Composed salads, such as the French classic Salade Niçoise, can be an entire summer meal. To create a composed salad, begin with lettuces or other greens placed on a platter. Then attractively arrange other

> **MISSION FOR THE DAY**
>
> Make a salad appropriate to the current season.

raw or cooked vegetables on top of the greens. Select seasonal produce, veggies your family enjoys, and ingredients that cover the color spectrum. The idea is to achieve an attractive array of colors and textures. Protein items (beans, fish, chicken) can be placed in the center or in strips across the top of the veggies to form a design. Final touches might include garnishes such as olives or capers scattered on top.

Chopped Salads Can Be a Complete Meal

In this salad concept, a range of veggies and other ingredients are chopped and tossed with a dressing. Again, these salads can be full meals in the summer. Add fish, chicken, meat, or whole grains to get added protein. Use lots of different colors for extra interest and nutrition.

Cruciferous Salads Are Rich with Nutrition and Texture

This salad combines one or more veggies in the cruciferous family, such as collards, kale, broccoli, Brussels sprouts, and cabbage. These fibrous vegetables work best shredded and then marinated in olive oil and lemon juice for about twenty minutes before serving, or in the case of cabbage, with various types of vinegar with oil.

feast on new salad possibilities

salads	variations		
composed salad variations	Arrange Boston lettuce leaves (1 to 2 heads) as cups for base of salad; grate 1 small beet, 1 carrot, 1 small turnip, and arrange in piles on the lettuce cups (2 cups per item provides nice color). Add some zucchini or bell pepper, tomato, and hard-boiled eggs. Dot with capers and olives and drizzle on lemony Niçoise dressing or your homemade favorite.	Arrange any flat leaf lettuce on a platter. Add the following in small piles arranged attractively over the lettuce: ¼ cup (50 g) marinated artichokes, grated red beet, grilled eggplant chunks, 1 cup (132 g) blanched cauliflower florets, smoked white fish or smoked oysters. Drizzle on lemony Niçoise dressing or your homemade favorite.	Arrange Boston lettuce (1 to 2 heads) as cups for base; add 1 cucumber, sliced and quartered; 1 cup (150 g) cherry tomatoes of all colors, sliced in half; 1 cup (150 g) sliced bell peppers in all colors; ¾ cup (75 g) tender green beans, blanched and cut in half; ⅓ cup (54 g) olives; dressing of 3 tablespoons (45 ml) olive oil, 2 tablespoons (8 g) fresh snipped dill, juice of 1 lemon, and salt to taste.
chopped salad variations	¾ pound (340 g) grilled chicken breasts and thighs cut into bite-size pieces, no bones; ½ head escarole; 8 prune plums, sliced; ¼ cup (36 g) almonds, chopped; red onion, sliced thinly; dressing of olive oil, balsamic vinegar, and sea salt to taste	2 ounces (55 g) thinly sliced pancetta; 1 red onion, sliced and caramelized; ½ an avocado; 30 grapes cut in half; ½ head chickory or escarole, shredded; toasted pine nuts, dressing of olive oil and lemon juice, and sea salt to taste	½ winter squash, cubed and parboiled; 1 red onion, sliced and caramelized; 1 orange, segmented with skin and peel removed; ½ bunch kale or Swiss chard leaves; ⅓ cup (33 g) walnuts, chopped; 3 ounces (85 g) crumbled goat cheese; dressing of olive oil, honey, red wine or sherry vinegar, and sea salt to taste
cruciferous salad variations	1 bunch kale (curly, lacinato, red Russian); ½ cup (55 g) chopped almonds; and dressing of juice of 1 lemon and 3 tablespoons (45 ml) extra-virgin olive oil; and salt to taste; fresh grana padano cheese grated on top	1 pound Brussels sprouts, cleaned and thinly sliced on a mandolin; dressing of ¼ cup (60 ml) olive oil and juice of 1 lemon; chopped almonds; grated pecorino cheese; salt and pepper to taste; add drained chick peas for more protein	½ head red cabbage, shredded; dressing of ¼ cup (60 ml) olive oil, 2 teaspoons (10 ml) cider vinegar, 1 tablespoon (15 ml) honey, and a couple drops of sesame oil; sprinkle of sunflower seeds on top; salt and pepper to taste

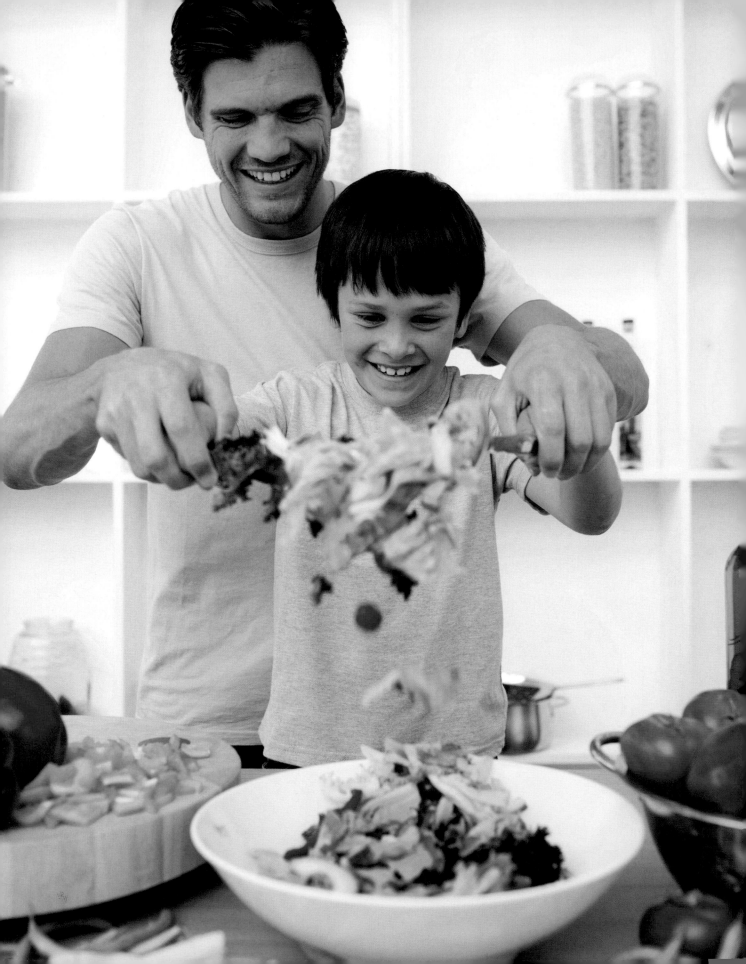

feast on new salad possibilities *continued*

salads	variations		
tomato salad variations	2 cups (300 g) cherry tomatoes of all colors, ½ tablespoon sweet or salty soy sauce, a few drops dark sesame oil, 1 tablespoon (8 g) toasted sesame seeds, ½ tablespoon olive oil, ¼ cup (4 g) chopped cilantro, and maybe some scallions	2 large green tomatoes, diced; ⅓ cup (50 g) sweet golden cherry tomatoes, halved; a few drops of pomegranate molasses; ¼ cup (36 g) chopped mint; 2 tablespoons (18 g) toasted pine nuts; olive oil and salt to taste	2 large sliced heirloom tomatoes, layered with 2 sliced hard-boiled eggs, basil (purple preferred), oregano, and capers; and dressing of fresh-squeezed orange juice, orange zest, and olive oil and grains of sea salt
bread salad variations	1 loaf dry, day-old bread, cubed; 2 ripe tomatoes, diced; 1 cucumber, diced; ½ red onion, minced; ⅓ cup (54 g) pitted olives; leaves from 4 sprigs fresh thyme; leaves from 10 springs fresh parsley; dressing of ¼ cup (60 ml) extra-virgin olive oil and 2 tablespoons (30 ml) red wine vinegar; 10 torn basil leaves as garnish; 1 can (15 ounces, or 420 g) chickpeas, drained and rinsed (optional)	1 loaf dry, day-old bread, cubed; 2 large heirloom tomatoes, diced; 2 cups (300 g) cubed watermelon; dressing of red wine vinegar and olive oil; basil cut into thin strips; feta cheese (optional); black olives	Cubed dry bread; ½ small butternut squash and 1 large beet, cubed and blanched; ⅓ bunch kale, sliced into shreds; ½ red onion, thinly sliced; 10 ounces (280 g) smoked mozzarella, cubed; leaves from 3 sprigs fresh thyme; dressing of olive oil, balsamic vinegar, grainy Dijon mustard, and salt and pepper

Enjoy Fresh Tomato Salads in Season

We mostly buy fresh local tomatoes—rather than supermarket ones—for salads. We feast on these during the months when tomatoes are in season. When the local crop is gone, we retire these recipes until the next time tomatoes come into season.

Bread Salads Are Practical and Fun to Fix

These are your go-to recipes when you have extra bread around the house—they're tasty, filling, and super easy to fix. Don't throw away delicious crusty bread because it's gotten hard. You can also use sliced bread you've frozen; just thaw it in the oven to toast it lightly, and then cut into cubes.

get started

Now that you've got the idea of how to work seasonally with our salad concepts, it's time to try them yourself:

- Select two or three salad concepts.
- Buy ingredients for two variations of each concept.
- Make one variation of each this week and a different variation of each next week.
- As a family, discuss and compare the results and your reactions.
- Ask family members to make suggestions for ingredient variations.

salad niçoise

This traditional favorite can easily be adapted to suit your family's preferences, what's seasonal, or what you have on hand.

8 new potatoes, with peels left on

½ pound (225 g) green beans

3 eggs

2 heads Boston lettuce

2 cans (5 ounces, or 140 g each) Italian tuna (packed in olive oil)

8 ounces (225 g) grape tomatoes

½ cup (50 g) Niçoise olives

3 tablespoons (26 g) capers

½ cup (120 ml) extra-virgin olive oil

1 lemon

3 sprigs fresh tarragon

6 leaves fresh basil

1 clove garlic

1 tablespoon (11 g) Dijon mustard

NOTE: *Children should use plastic or table knives for all child steps that require cutting or chopping.*

ADULT Fill a medium saucepan halfway with water, add the potatoes, and bring to boil over high heat.

CHILD Trim the ends of the green beans and cut in half.

ADULT Blanch the green beans in the boiling water for 2 minutes, (or microwave, covered with a damp paper towel, on High for 3 minutes). Remove with a slotted spoon.

ADULT & CHILD Drop the eggs gently into the same boiling water and cook for 15 minutes. Remove with a slotted spoon. Cool and remove shells.

ADULT Check the potatoes periodically, and remove them when a fork can go in easily but they are not mushy. Cool.

CHILD Wash and dry the lettuce. Arrange leaves attractively on a large platter, so the leaves cover the platter and fan out around the edges.

ADULT & CHILD Open the cans of tuna (adult removes the sharp lid). Drain and flake tuna with a fork into a small bowl. Place tuna in the center of the platter.

CHILD Cut the grape tomatoes and eggs in half; arrange around the tuna.

CHILD Peel the cooled potatoes, and cut them into quarters; arrange them decoratively on the platter.

CHILD Measure the olives and capers; sprinkle over the salad.

CHILD Add the green beans in small bunches around the platter.

ADULT & CHILD Measure the olive oil in a large measuring cup.

CHILD Squeeze the lemon into the cup with the oil.

CHILD Chop the tarragon and basil, and add them to the cup.

CHILD Mince the garlic and measure the mustard, and add them to the cup. Whisk together until well combined. Drizzle the dressing evenly over the entire salad.

PREP TIME	COOK TIME	YIELD
20 minutes	15 minutes	10 servings

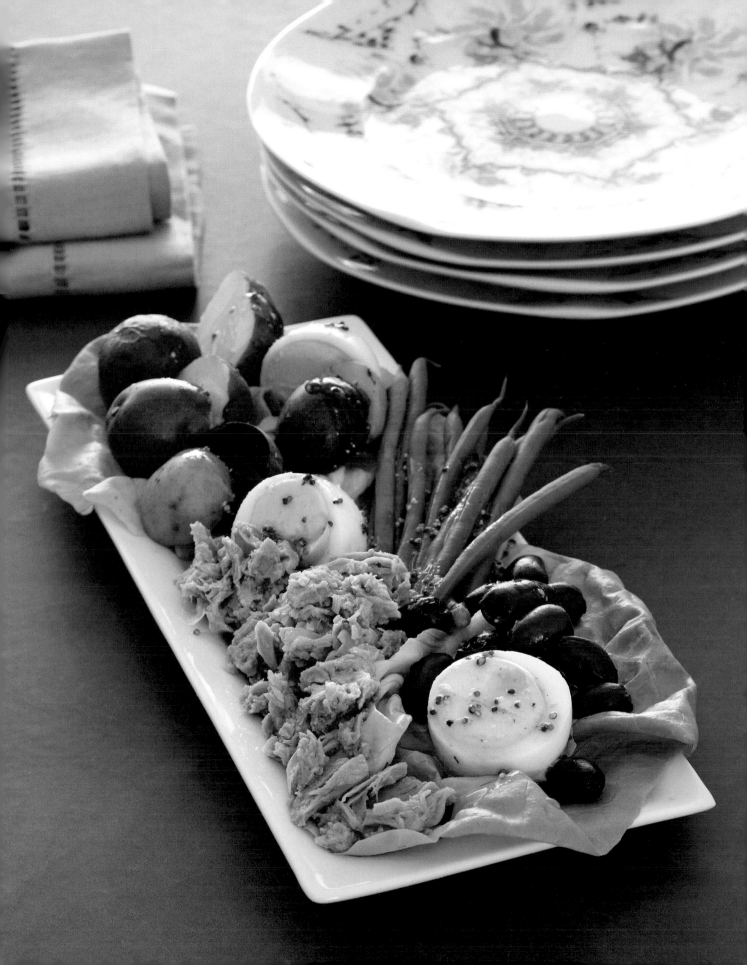

{ DAY 16 } Switch to Whole Grains

FOR MORE THAN 8,000 YEARS, whole grains have provided our bodies with a healthy, efficient, and inexpensive source of energy. But in the last half century, packaged foods containing highly refined grains (e.g., instant rice, instant oatmeal, chips, and crackers) have become a multi-billion-dollar industry. Eating refined grains gives us short-term energy, but not a longer-term sense of fullness after the meal is finished. Hence, our bodies crave more calories because we're not getting enough sustained nutrition—and weight gain is the unwanted consequence.

Whole grains are much healthier, and the good news is they have become more available in recent years. The bad news is many whole-grain products are too highly processed. Packaged foods that contain whole grains may be riddled with unwanted ingredients, such as sugar and preservatives. It takes skill to identify true, unadulterated whole grains from the impostors, but you can buy an exciting variety of traditional whole grains in packages or bulk. Add these grains to your family meals for a tasty shot of super nutrition.

whole grains help protect against many chronic diseases

Grains contain a key source of energy known as carbohydrates. Like legumes, grains are the edible seeds of various plants. The term "whole grain" means they aren't stripped of fibrous bran (exterior) and

MISSION FOR THE DAY

Try a whole grain you've never eaten before.

germ, which contain the greatest concentrations of B vitamins, minerals, phytochemicals, and protein.

An article in *Nutrition Research Reviews* reported on a review of multiple studies and found that whole grains helped protect against cancer, cardiovascular disease, diabetes, obesity, and other chronic diseases. The Centers for Disease Control and Prevention reported that in 2008 one-third of children and adolescents in the United States were overweight or obese, and that trend is growing at an alarming rate, putting more and more kids at risk for these illnesses.

The fiber in whole grains slows the absorption of carbohydrates in the body, providing sustained energy. It also protects the delicate wall of the intestines as it pushes food through your digestive system and stabilizes bowel regularity.

Buy the most unadulterated whole-grain products. Consider trying whole grains other than wheat. Just as eating a variety of fruits and vegetables can be approached as a multisensory adventure, so can exploring the various flavors and textures of whole grains. Most cultures have traditionally used delicious whole grains for flavor and health in their cuisines, and here is a peek at some to inspire you!

10 easy strategies to add whole grains to your family's diet

grain	origins and characteristics	contemporary use
amaranth	South America	Higher-quality protein than wheat, high in calcium and vitamins A and C Cook like rice and use similarly; serve with stew or curry
barley	Ancient Egypt	Becomes creamy when cooked slowly; can take longer than rice to cook Add to soups; substitute for rice in risotto; cook like rice and mix with a variety of ingredients for a healthy salad
buckwheat	Northern Europe	Used whole as groats or ground into flour; nutty flavor Groats cook like rice; add flour to pancakes or crepes—check recipes for ratio of buckwheat to regular flour so you get the consistency you want
corn	Central Mexico	Stone-ground offers the most fiber and flavor Substitute corn for flour tortillas; use stone-ground grits; add cornmeal to muffins; use in polentas
millet	Africa	Contains 16 to 22 percent protein vs. wheat's 10 percent Choose millet flour for gluten-free diets; cook as pilaf and combine with veggies
oats	Middle East	Find as rolled or steel cut Cook steel cut or rolled for hot porridge; add rolled to cookies, muffins, pancakes, and waffles; grind and use instead of flour when breading fish or for fried green tomatoes
quinoa	Peru	High in protein; nutty flavor; beautiful red and white varieties Substitute for rice or oatmeal; prepare with chopped veggies and dressing for healthy salads
rice	Southeast Asia	Choose the least processed: jasmine, arborio, and brown basmati
rye	Near East	Denser and darker than whole wheat due to protein structure Look for artisan breads made with rye four
wheat	Near East	Whole wheat bulgur and couscous Choose whole wheat artisan breads; substitute whole wheat flour for white in recipes (use about 50 percent of each type of flour for optimal elasticity and texture)

People with celiac disease can benefit from eating a gluten-free diet that includes various nutritious grains. They should avoid three grains that contain gluten—wheat, barley, and rye—and be careful with commercially processed oats that can contain gluten.

- Scandinavians eat rye "crisp bread" in the morning with butter and cheese.
- Mexicans enjoy stone-ground corn tortillas as their daily bread.
- The Japanese eat soba noodles made from buckwheat.
- The Swiss eat muesli, which contains rolled oats.

get started

Try one of these easy strategies to add more delicious whole grains to your family's diet:

- Add barley to both homemade and canned soups for greater texture, flavor, and nutrition.
- Experiment with barley, quinoa, buckwheat, and steel-cut oats for breakfast.
- Swap brown basmati for white rice in recipes; sprinkle with some cumin—delicious!
- Experiment with multigrain breads and muffins; some very dark types include molasses and their slight sweetness can make them more palatable to children.
- Add rolled oats to most cookie and muffin recipes; with all the whole-grain flours available, you can keep experimenting until you find one your family likes best.
- Experiment to find your family's favorite brand of whole wheat pasta.
- Serve creamy or baked polenta under stew or as a side dish; top with a bit of grated parmesan cheese for extra taste.
- Prepare whole-grain pilafs, such as barley, with diced veggies and a homemade dressing; add seafood or cubed chicken for a complete and delicious meal.

date nut bars

This old-world recipe from Lynn's grandmother is a delicious and healthy sweet treat.

1 pound (455 g) pitted dates

1 cup (200 g) granulated sugar

½ cup (120 ml) water

1 cup (100 g) walnuts

1 cup (225 g) butter

1 cup (225 g) packed brown sugar

½ cup (120 ml) warm water

1 teaspoon baking soda

2½ cups (248 g) flour

2½ cups (200 g) rolled oats

2 tablespoons (16 g) confectioner's sugar, for garnish

ADDITIONAL COOKING EQUIPMENT: Electric mixer, 13 x 9 x 2-inch (33 x 23 x 5 cm) baking pan

NOTE: *Children should use plastic or table knives for all child steps that require cutting or chopping.*

ADULT Preheat the oven to 350°F (180°C, or gas mark 4).

CHILD Cut the pitted dates in half and place them in a small saucepan.

ADULT & CHILD Measure granulated sugar and the ½ cup (120 ml) water and add to the saucepan. Cook over medium heat, stirring occasionally, until dates are soft.

ADULT Determine when dates are done by observing whether they are beginning to lose their shape when pressed with a wooden spoon. Remove from heat.

CHILD Meanwhile, help chop walnuts coarsely. Add the nuts to the softened dates and set aside to cool.

ADULT & CHILD Measure the butter and brown sugar into a large mixing bowl, and mix with an electric mixer until smooth. Measure the ½ cup (120 ml) warm water into a small bowl and add the baking soda; stir until dissolved. Add flour and the baking soda mixture to the creamed butter and sugar. Mix well.

CHILD Measure the rolled oats and fold it into the batter, stirring until mixed thoroughly. Butter the baking pan.

ADULT & CHILD Spread one-half of the batter in an even layer over the bottom of the baking pan. Using a wooden spoon, spread the date-nut filling evenly over the batter (moisten the spoon with water if mixture is too sticky to spread). Spread the rest of the batter over the filling—you can do this with your clean hands.

ADULT Bake in preheated oven for 40 to 45 minutes, or until golden brown. Cut into squares and dust with confectioner's sugar.

PREP TIME	COOK TIME	YIELD
20 minutes	40 to 45 minutes	about 3 dozen bars

scandinavian barley salad with apples

Enjoy this recipe for lunch or a light dinner. Mussels are an inexpensive and highly nutritious shellfish that children usually come to enjoy because of their gentle taste. Giving children an opportunity to help clean the mussels piques their curiosity to eat them.

1 cup (200 g) pearl barley

1 large carrot

1 medium turnip

½ bunch fresh dill

1 pound (455 g) mussels

2 cups (475 ml) vegetable or chicken broth

1 small red onion

1 medium apple (Golden Delicious, preferably)

¼ cup (60 ml) extra-virgin olive oil

1 tablespoon (15 ml) apple cider vinegar

Sea salt and freshly ground pepper

Smoked paprika

ADDITIONAL COOKING EQUIPMENT:
Apple corer and segmenter (optional)

NOTE: *Children should use plastic or table knives for all child steps that require cutting or chopping.*

ADULT Fill a saucepan with 2½ cups (591 ml) water and bring to boil. Add barley, reduce heat, and simmer 15 to 20 minutes, or until tender.

CHILD While the barley is simmering, scrub the carrot and turnip.

ADULT Slice the unpeeled carrots crosswise into 2 sections. Slice each section in half lengthwise, and these halves lengthwise again. You will have 8 lengths of carrot.

CHILD Line up 2 to 3 carrot lengths and slice them crosswise. Continue until the entire carrot is diced. Add to a large mixing bowl.

ADULT & CHILD Adult cuts the turnip into thin slices. Child cuts each turnip slice into thin strips, rotates the strips, and cuts them into a small, even dice. Add to the bowl.

CHILD Snip the dill into the mixing bowl with kitchen shears.

ADULT Clean the mussels well, removing the "barb" or stringy part. Make sure they are closed or closing to ensure they have not perished before cooking. Place second saucepan over medium heat.

ADULT & CHILD Measure and pour broth into second saucepan. Carefully add the mussels and simmer over medium heat about 10 minutes, or until each mussel opens wide.

ADULT Dice the red onion finely and add to the mixing bowl. Peel the apple; core and cut, or use segmenter, into 8 segments.

CHILD Slice the apple segments in half lengthwise, and then help slice each length into thin slices and add to the bowl.

ADULT When the barley is tender, drain and add to the veggies.

CHILD Help measure the oil and vinegar. Add to the bowl. Mix well.

ADULT Remove cooled mussels from their shells and add to the barley mixture. Mix again gently. Season to taste with salt and pepper. Serve each portion with a dusting of smoked paprika.

PREP TIME	COOK TIME	YIELD
15 to 20 minutes	10 minutes	6 to 8 servings

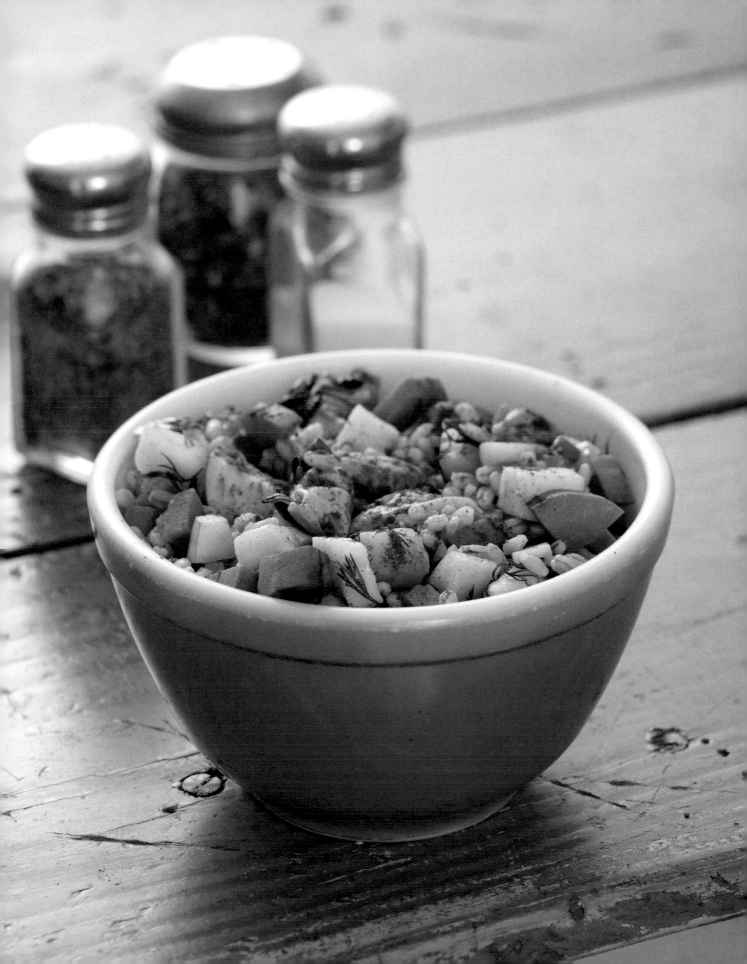

{DAY 17} Serve More Legumes

MANY CULTURES throughout the world rely on legumes as a regular source of essential nutrients. Legumes are nutritious, versatile, economical, seasonless, and sustainable foods. These are compelling reasons to serve more of these plant-based foods to your family. The legumes we use in our recipes include beans, peas, and lentils, and we're sure you'll find them anything but dull.

What about the kids, you wonder? Will they eat legumes? Fear not. Time and again we have watched children who claim they don't like beans devour Persian Spring Soup with lentils, kidney beans, and garbanzos. Kids love to be surprised! As they make the soup together and taste how delicious it is, they become eager to try other recipes with legumes from other cultures. In "Look Who's Cooking," our elementary program, children plant several different kinds of beans that are featured in the recipes from various cultures. They rush to school each day to watch the transformation from a seemingly inert seed to a living thing with tiny leaves that grow bigger by the hour.

legumes provide the health benefits of veggies and grains, plus protein

A scientific review published in the *British Medical Journal* in 2008 revealed that the Mediterranean-type diet—high in legumes and low in meat—is best for a healthy heart and body. Legumes are distinguished by their fruit, which grows in the form of a pod

and contains seeds. All legumes are seeds. That means they are packed with all the nutrients necessary to create an entire new plant.

Legumes have plenty to offer nutritionally. They're naturally low in fat and rich in vitamins, including folic acid, and minerals such as copper, magnesium, and iron, as well as phytochemicals.

Legumes, like whole grains, contain carbohydrates as well as soluble and insoluble fiber. Soluble fiber helps reduce the "bad" LDL cholesterol in the blood and can lower the risk of heart disease. It also slows down carbohydrate absorption and prevents unwanted spikes in blood glucose levels. Insoluble fiber enhances water absorption in the colon, which helps prevent constipation and digestive problems.

Legumes also contribute plant-based protein. The United States Department of Agriculture (USDA) includes legumes in the "protein" category on MyPlate, which shows how to use the five food groups to create a balanced diet. Most vegetarians eat plenty of legumes to get the protein and iron nonvegetarians consume in meat, fowl, and fish. Add a little vitamin C in the form of tomatoes, and you'll dramatically increase the amount of iron your body can absorb from the legumes.

8 great legume ideas from around the world

country or region	legume	dish
north and south america	Red kidney beans	Chili: the American favorite made with ground beef, onion, garlic, beans, and chili powder
china	Soybeans (tofu), fermented black beans	Stir-fry: with tofu or sauce made with fermented black beans
ecuador	Pinto beans, lentils	Menestra de Porotos: pinto bean stew
egypt	Fava beans, chickpeas	Hummus and falafel: from chickpeas Ful: mashed fava beans, for breakfast
italy	White beans, peas, fava beans, chickpeas, lentils	Pasta Fazul: soup with small macaroni, bits of meat and veggies, and white beans Rizi Bizi: risotto with fresh green peas and herbs
iran	Lentils, red kidney beans, fava beans, chickpeas	Lentil and raisin polo: steamed rice, lentils, raisins, and cinnamon Baghali polo: steamed rice, chicken, lima beans, and dill
mexico	Black beans, pinto beans	Frijoles negros: stewed black beans with oil and epazote Enchiladas: stewed beans with cheese, rolled in tortillas
west africa	Black-eyed peas or "cow peas"	Stew with black-eyed peas, onion, ginger, tomato, and spices

Many people consider legumes a meat substitute. But this sells legumes short because they also provide fiber, folic acid, and phytochemicals. Fiber, which is not found in meat, is particularly important for digestive health and the feeling the fullness. Fiber occurs naturally in legumes, making them a better choice than processed foods that add fiber artificially. If you're unsure how much fiber your children need, check the American Heart Association's chart that offers guidance by age.

economical legumes help you save money

Industrialized countries such as the United States have instituted factory-style methods in meat production. Yet, raising animals for food can require more energy, land, and water and causes more pollution than raising plants. Additionally, many producers inject animals with hormones to make them grow more quickly and add antibiotics to animals' feed to control diseases. Eating fish can pose problems, too, as pollution in the oceans and waterways can contaminate aquatic creatures. By serving your family more legumes, you can reduce some of the potential health risks associated with eating meat, fowl, or fish.

Beans, peas, and lentils are also inexpensive, especially when dried. Making them a bigger part of your family's diet can reduce your grocery bill. Consider cutting down the amount of meat in soups and stews, and adding legumes. These dishes can be flavorful, satisfying, and nutritional. You can use the money you save to buy higher quality meat (grass-fed, organic, hormone and antibiotic free) and leaner cuts that let you lower the amount of saturated fat in your diet.

multicultural recipes offer a delicious change at mealtime

Traditional dishes from other cultures often feature legumes. These dishes offer a delicious change from meatloaf, hamburger, barbecue, roasts, and meat-based casseroles. In our programs, we win over children by telling stories about legumes' nutritional and cultural significance. In many cultures, for instance, legumes symbolize spring and birth. When kids learn about colorful connections with food, they grow curious; legumes cease being small, hard, dry objects and become something magical.

For inspiration, take a look at the chart on the previous page for examples of diverse dishes from around the world.

get started

By adding legumes to stews, soups, salads, rice dishes, and meat-based casseroles—as well as eating them for snacks—you help your family get a healthy ratio of plant-to-animal protein. Here are some ideas to get you started:

- Add legumes, hot or cold, to your favorite recipes to boost nutrition.
- Add canned beans in salads.
- Try a new after-school snack: Buy a package of edamame, boil them, and serve them warm in the pods with kosher salt. Place a pod in your mouth and use your teeth to pop it open. Eat the seeds and discard the empty pod. Delicious!

You can adapt the yummy legume recipes we provide to the different seasons. Seasonal variations keep your family's meals fresh and interesting.

black-eyed pea and collard soup

This is a traditional soul food combination. Rather than cooking it for hours, we transform the ingredients into a lovely soup while maintaining their flavor and texture. The golden beets add a burst of sweetness and color.

1 pound (455 g) dried black-eyed peas

1 large onion

1 pound (455 g) ham steak

1 tablespoon (15 ml) olive oil

½ bunch collard greens, about 6 cups (400 g), chopped

8 cups (1.9 L) water

1 teaspoon salt

1 very large golden beet

Salt and freshly ground black pepper

Vietnamese Sriracha hot sauce (optional)

NOTE: *Children should use plastic or table knives for all child steps that require cutting or chopping.*

ADULT Soak the peas in a bowl overnight, adding more water as needed so they can become reconstituted.

ADULT When you are ready to make the soup, chop the onion into an even dice.

ADULT & CHILD On a separate cutting board with a separate knife, dice the ham steak into ½-inch (13 mm) cubes.

ADULT Heat a stockpot over high heat and add the oil.

ADULT & CHILD Add the ham and stir and cook 5 minutes, or until browned. Add the onions, lower the heat, and cook 5 to 8 minutes, or until softened.

CHILD Meanwhile, slice the collard leaves into ribbons, about 1 inch (2.5 cm) wide. When the onions have softened, add the collard and cook over high heat until they turn bright green and collapse and soften.

ADULT & CHILD Drain the black-eyed peas and add to the stockpot.

ADULT & CHILD Add 8 cups (1.9 L) water and the 1 teaspoon salt, and bring to a boil. Turn heat to and simmer for 10 minutes.

ADULT Meanwhile, scrub the golden beet but do not peel. Fill a saucepan with water and bring to a boil. Chop the beet into a ½-inch (13 mm) dice. Blanch in the boiling water for 2 to 3 minutes, or until slightly softened and no longer crunchy. Remove beets with slotted spoon and add to the soup. Season to taste with salt and pepper.

ADULT Serve with a drizzle of Sriracha to add a kick!

PREP TIME	COOK TIME	YIELD
15 minutes	30 minutes	6 to 8 servings

merche's white bean and chorizo spanish stew

Mercedes grew up eating this dish, and she loves making it with freshly shelled beans. Her children love to shell the beans, and fresh beans make it quicker to prepare than using dry ones.

½ yellow onion

½ red or yellow bell pepper

1 small zucchini

2 cloves garlic

½ pound (225 g) Spanish chorizo sausage or Portuguese linguica sausage (do not use Mexican or Caribbean sausage)

4 to 5 tablespoons (60 to 75 ml) extra-virgin Spanish olive oil

3 sprigs fresh thyme

4 cups (946 ml) water

2 cans (15 ounces, or 430 g each) white beans, rinsed and drained

Salt and pepper

NOTE: *Children should use plastic or table knives for all child steps that require cutting or chopping.*

ADULT Slice the onion.

CHILD Dice the onion slices.

ADULT Slice the bell pepper and zucchini.

CHILD Dice the bell pepper and zucchini slices.

ADULT Smash the garlic cloves with the flat side of a chef's knife to remove the peel and slice thinly. Cut the chorizo into slices about ¼ inch (6 mm) thick.

CHILD Help mince the garlic slices.

ADULT Heat a large stockpot over medium heat. Add the olive oil and the onion and bell pepper, and cook, stirring often. When the onion becomes translucent, add the zucchini, garlic, and chorizo slices. Cook over medium heat for 5 to 8 minutes, or until the chorizo is browned. Add more olive oil if needed.

ADULT & CHILD Remove thyme leaves from the stems and add to the stockpot. Measure the 4 cups (946 ml) water and add to the stockpot. Add the beans.

ADULT Bring to a boil, lower heat, and simmer 15 more minutes. Season to taste with salt and pepper, and serve.

PREP TIME	COOK TIME	YIELD
5 minutes	15 minutes	4 servings

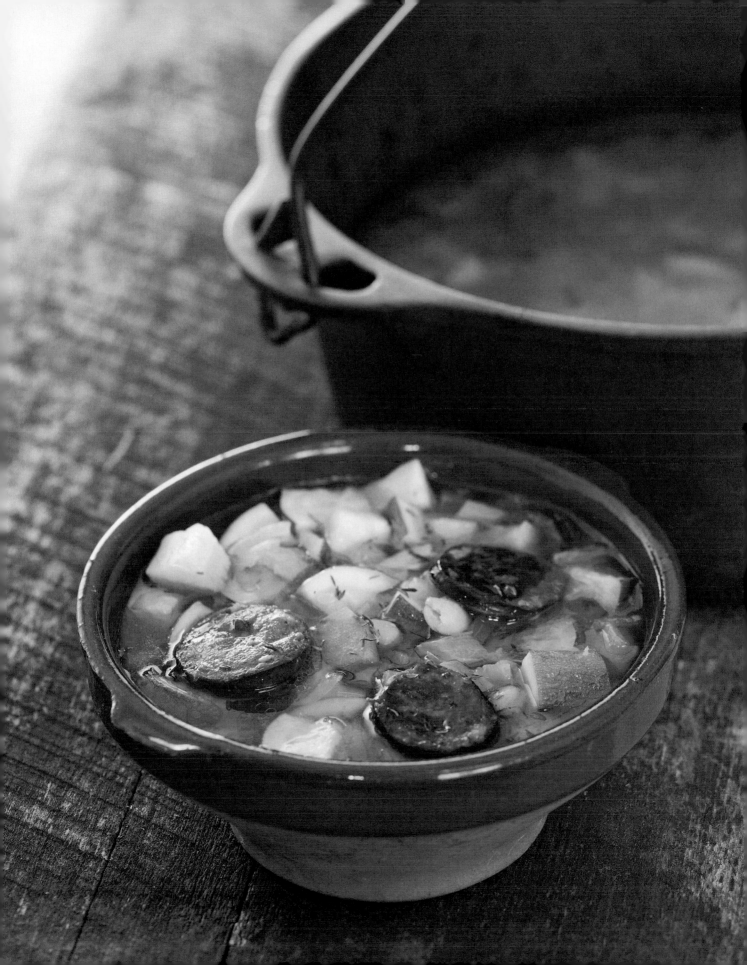

{DAY 18} Make Whole Food Snacks a Priority

SNACKING HAS GOTTEN A BAD RAP. In recent decades, as junk food became synonymous with snack food, it became hard to see the benefits of snacks. In truth, snacks—or mini-meals between main meals—are an important part of a healthy diet. They can nutritionally balance and complete other meals, and provide energy between meals. When the school day ends, kids are hungry. Without snacks, they probably would not sustain their energy between lunch at school and dinner. Even adults often need something to keep them going between meals.

The amount of food children need for a snack depends on how much they ate at the previous meal and when their next meal will be. How active or inactive they are during the day is also a factor.

play snack food detective with your children

On Day 7 you learned to play the game we call "Food Detective." You can play this game with your children to give them a better understanding of the snacks they eat. Many snacks are really no better than candy, offering no nutrition. Go to the supermarket with your kids and choose a favorite snack, and then examine it according to the list of questions given in that chapter.

MISSION FOR THE DAY

Offer only whole food snacks to your family.

Children's hunger may vary on cold or hot days, or if they are in the middle of a growth spurt. Usually, children are quite capable of knowing how much they need to eat. However, *what* they snack on and *how often* have changed in recent years.

A review study conducted by the University of North Carolina in 2010 found that in the past three decades children have significantly increased the amount of snacks they ate and hence the amount of calories. The largest calorie increase occurred among children between ages two and six, indicating that unhealthy eating patterns start at an early age. Salty snacks, candy, sweetened beverages, and increased portion sizes were the major calorie contributors in snacks.

Highly processed snacks don't offer much of a satiating effect, meaning kids have to eat more to feel full. In sum, children are loading up on high-calorie junk foods that contain little or no nutritional value. Nature provides many delicious foods that are ideal, nutritious choices for between-meal snacks. The following short, multicultural chart gives a few examples.

whole food snacks from across the globe	
country or region	**snack foods**
united states	Banana bread, bran muffins, fruit juice, oatmeal cookies, peanut butter sandwich, popcorn, trail mix nuts, yogurt with fruit
india	Breads, samosa, lentil and other vegetable dips
greece	Figs, hummus, olives, stuffed grape leaves, whole wheat pita, yogurt dip
japan	Edamame, dried fish and squid, mocha, red beans, rice crackers, sweet potato chips, wasabi peas
egypt	Eggplant dip, fava beans, hummus, roasted watermelon seeds, whole wheat pita
iran	Almonds and salt, cucumber and salt, fava beans with vinegar and spices, roasted corn on the cob, yogurt dip
italy	Crostini (bread with cheese and veggie toppings), breadsticks with parma ham, olives
spain	Bocadillo (baked bread with cheese, ham, chorizo, or chocolate), sunflower seeds, toasted corn kernels
scandinavia	Flatbread with sliced cheese
mexico	Salsa and cheeses with tortillas, tropical fruits
caribbean	Plantains, tropical fruits, yucca chips

choose nutrient-rich snacks to satisfy hunger

Ideally, snacks should contribute vitamins, minerals, phytochemicals, carbohydrates, fiber, proteins, and healthy fats to your diet. These essential nutrients keep children, especially adolescents, more satisfied between meals than empty calories can. Here are some tips to help you plan for nutritious snacks:

♡ Plan ahead for snacks.
♡ Read food labels when purchasing prepared products.
♡ Think of sweet treats as mini-desserts—serve to give a little excitement to an already nutritionally satisfied child, but don't offer them to satisfy hunger.

Modern parents face a challenge. Many children go to after-school activities and don't arrive home until dinnertime. How can you make sure they eat healthy snacks? Here is a list of portable, healthy, and homemade snacks to complete your children's diet:

♡ **fruits and vegetables:** fresh fruit; cut-up veggies and hummus in a container; cherry tomatoes (vary the colors)
♡ **whole grains:** multigrain or whole-grain crackers without added sodium; sandwiches made with whole-grain breads
♡ **nuts and seeds:** homemade trail mix combining nuts and dried fruit
♡ **dairy products:** cheese and yogurt in child-friendly sizes and options; unsweetened yogurt with honey added
♡ **sweets:** provided only as afternoon treats

whole foods in a snap

snack	how to prepare
apple and honey	Cut and place apple segments on a plate. Squeeze some honey into a corner of a plastic bag. Twist to close. Cut the tip off the corner to make a tiny hole. Invite children to squeeze out the honey, drizzling it in a pretty pattern. (Note: Use different colored apples and leave the skins on.)
fruit salad	Select seasonal fruits (substitute thawed frozen ones in winter) and peel, slice, or cut into bite-size pieces. Place in a large bowl. Squeeze half a lime over the fruit and drizzle with 1 tablespoon (20 g) honey. Stir well and serve.
pastina and cheese	Grate a small amount (⅓ cup, or 42 g) of cheddar, pecorino, or other mild-tasting cheese. Cook ¾ cup (75 g) pastina and put in a bowl. Add the grated cheese and 1 to 2 tablespoons (15 to 30 ml) of milk. Add diced raw veggies or grated carrot as well.
kebobs	Cube cheese and fruit, making sure you have roughly equal quantities of each item. Have children use coffee stirrers as skewers to make snack kebobs, selecting patterns (e.g., 1 strawberry half, 2 cheese cubes, and 1 grape. Repeat.). Dip into yogurt dressing.
cherry tomatoes	Mix chopped chives or basil into ½ cup (125 g) ricotta cheese (part skim is fine). Season to taste with salt and pepper. Cut cherry or grape tomatoes in half. Have children scoop out the seeds from the tomatoes using a small spoon. Replace seeds with the cheese mixture.
nut butter crunch	Spread nut butter on flatbread (try cashew or pumpkin seed butter for amazing flavor and a burst of energy).
banana crunch	Mash 1 large (or 2 small) very ripe bananas (children will love this step). Mix ¼ to ⅓ cup (30 to 40 g) granola into mashed banana. Spread onto thin flatbread wafers.
spiced pepitas	For preschool children, add the following to a small saucepan: 1 tablespoon (14 g) butter, 2 tablespoons (30 g) packed brown sugar, and 2 teaspoons (5 g) ground cumin. Heat on low until the butter melts. Add 3 cups (420 g) pepitas and stir well to coat.
applesauce	Peel and segment 6 or more apples. Place in a stockpot and add water to about half the height of the apples. Add 3 tablespoons (39 g) sugar and 2 teaspoons (5 g) cinnamon. Cook over medium heat, stirring as needed until apples soften.
flower sandwich	Cut whole-grain or pumpernickel-raisin bread slices into quarters. Spread with nut butter, herb butter, chèvre or ricotta cheese (with a bit of honey added). Sprinkle with fresh arugula and edible flower petals from your garden, such as pansy, nasturtium, geranium, marigold, or rose.
trail mix	Place the following in separate bowls: cheerios, pumpkin seeds, walnut pieces, tiny pretzels, raisins, banana chips, and other dried fruit in small pieces. Place spoons in each bowl and give children plastic bags to put a spoonful of each into their bags.
avocado crunch	Mash 1 or 2 ripe avocados. Squeeze in juice ½ lemon, and add 2 teaspoons (8 g) flaxseeds. Add a pinch of salt. Top onto cucumber disks and dust with sweet paprika.

{DAY 19} Dress Up Fruit for Desserts

IF YOU ARE NOT ALREADY A FRUIT LOVER, we're going do our best to convert you. In our homes, we set out fresh fruit in bowls in several readily accessible places, and it gets eaten quickly. Only perishable berries are kept in the fridge. We try to buy as much as we can from the local farmers' market and choose organic when we can afford it. Check www.ewg.org to find the Environmental Working Group's "Dirty Dozen" and "Clean 15" lists for more information about buying healthy produce.

MISSION FOR THE DAY

Select a family member to be in charge of planning and preparing a simple fruit dessert for dinner.

adapt lynn's apple pie with seasonal fruits

I love pies with soft, voluptuous fillings, so I devised the method of prepping the apples—explained in my following apple pie recipe—to achieve the texture and depth of flavor my family loves. My sons beg for the pie throughout the fall, and I probably make it seven or eight times each year. I've even converted some serious cooks to this recipe! Seasonal variations are easy—mixed berries, berries with rhubarb, pitted cherries, or sliced stone fruit. Use ¼ cup (50 g) sugar (more if fruit is tart) and 2 tablespoons (12 g) flour or tapioca to absorb the juices released during baking. Make the bottom crust and pour in the desired filling, add the top crust, and you're done—no need to sauté the fruit first; I only do that when I'm using apples.

We also celebrate the seasons by making fresh fruit the star of simple desserts, just as previous generations did. We want our families to think of dessert as a ripe and luscious seasonal fruit, not some synthetic sugary concoction. As parents, we are giving our children healthy habits for life. Rather than the empty calories of cake and cookies, a piece of fruit or fruit-based dessert offers nutrition as well as a sweet treat at the end of a meal.

Here are some simple ideas that you can use to make fruit a festive dessert.

⏱ get started

Select a fruit you rarely eat and make a simple dessert around it:

- ♡ Use chocolate fondue or serve sliced fruit with sweetened ricotta cheese and lemon (see chart on page 129).
- ♡ Have a tropical fruit discovery feast—buy an array of tropical fruits and slice them on a plate or platter. Explore and compare their colors, flavors, degrees of sweetness and tartness, noting your family's preferences.

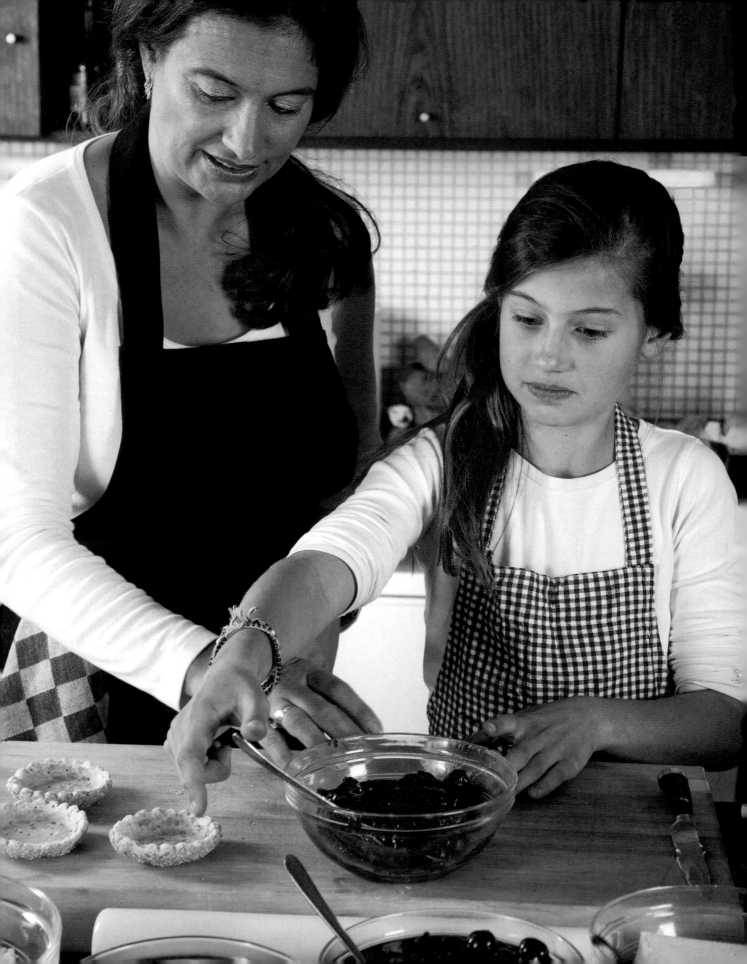

how to transform fruit into delicious desserts

dessert	method
dessert crepes	Make a crepe batter and sprinkle sugar, a few drops of lemon juice, and some stewed fresh or dried fruit inside (use jam if you are in a rush).
fruit fondue	Cut up one or an array of fresh seasonal fruits, keeping the peel when edible; dip fruit into delectable melted dark chocolate.
fruit fool	Blend fresh berries or currents in food processor until just crushed. Add a bit of sugar so mixture is not too tart. Whip cream with little or no sugar, swirl into the fruit—streaks are fine. Garnish with a whole berry.
ricotta and fresh fruit	Whip 1 cup (250 g) fresh ricotta cheese (whole or part skim) with an electric mixture. Add confectioner's sugar to taste (about 1 tablespoon, or 8 g) and a squeeze of fresh lemon juice. Slice fresh fruit and serve with a dollop of the whipped ricotta.
rustic fruit tart	Make a recipe for a 1-crust pie crust. Roll out the dough onto a baking sheet. In a bowl, make a fruit filling of your favorite seasonal fruit(s), and then toss with sugar and a bit of flour or tapioca to absorb the juices. Place the fruit in the center of the pie crust and fold up the edges 2 to 3 inches (5 to 7.5 cm) all around, leaving 4 to 5 inches (10 to 13 cm) of fruit visible in the center. Bake as you would a fruit pie.
zabaglione	This fluffy and delicious Italian egg yolk mixture is a fascinating food science lesson for children. The yolks transform into mounds of soft clouds. It begs for a fruit accompaniment—explore your favorite combinations.

lynn's signature apple pie

Lynn's apple pie is famous among her lucky family and friends, who have been converted to her method of sautéing the apples with cinnamon and a small amount of sugar before baking. Make it once and you'll be converted, too!

FOR THE FILLING:

8 to 10 medium to large apples (mixture of tart and sweet varieties)

3 tablespoons (42 g) unsalted butter

⅓ cup (63 g) sugar (less if apples are sweet)

1½ teaspoons cinnamon

FOR THE CRUST:

1¾ cup (174 g) flour (you can use up to ¾ cup [98 g] whole wheat)

1 teaspoon kosher or sea salt

10 tablespoons (143 g) butter

⅓ cup (80 ml) ice water (less if it is very humid or warm)

1 egg

2 tablespoons (30 g) turbinado sugar

ADDITIONAL COOKING EQUIPMENT:
Pastry cutter (optional), pastry brush, rolling pin, and 9-inch (23-cm) pie pan

NOTE: *Children should use plastic or table knives for all child steps that require cutting or chopping.*

TO MAKE THE FILLING:

ADULT & CHILD Peel, core, and segment the apples.

ADULT Melt the butter in a large skillet over medium heat. Add the apples and sauté.

ADULT & CHILD Measure the sugar and cinnamon. Add to the apples and mix well. Stir and cook 6 to 10 minutes, or until the apples are softened and browned. Remove from heat and cool. Set aside.

TO MAKE THE CRUST AND BAKE:

ADULT Preheat oven to 375°F (190°C, or gas mark 5).

CHILD Help measure the flour and salt in a large mixing bowl. Mix well.

CHILD Help cut butter into small pieces and scatter over flour mixture.

ADULT & CHILD Cut the butter into the flour using pastry cutter or your fingertips until you have small pieces.

ADULT Add just enough ice water so dough forms into a ball. Chill 30 minutes.

ADULT & CHILD Cut dough into 2 pieces. Put 1 piece back in refrigerator and roll out the other half to about 1 inch (2.5 cm) larger than your pie pan. Place into the pie pan leaving edges ragged.

ADULT Roll out the second piece of dough to the same size as the first. Spoon cooled filling into the pie pan. Place the second piece of dough over the filling. Pinch edges together to form an even edge.

CHILD Cut 3 to 4 tiny diamond-shaped vents in a design on the top.

ADULT Beat the egg in a small bowl. Using a pastry brush, brush the egg over the top of the crust. Sprinkle with the turbinado sugar.

ADULT Bake in preheated oven about 40 minutes.

PREP TIME	COOK TIME	YIELD
20 minutes	40 minutes	1 double-crusted pie

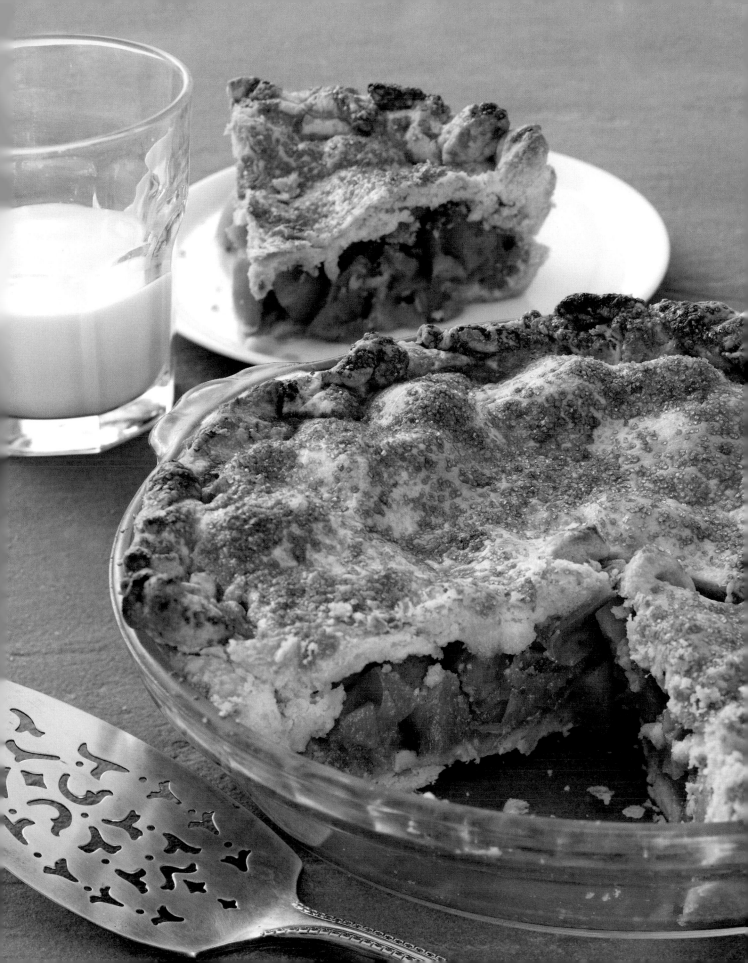

zabaglione with fruit

This fluffy dessert is fantastic with fresh berries or stone fruit. In the winter, use drained and thawed frozen berries.

5 jumbo eggs

½ cup (120 ml) marsala, cream sherry, or other sweet wine

3 ounces (84 g) sugar

Pinch of salt

1 cup (145 g) berries

ADDITIONAL COOKING EQUIPMENT: Electric hand mixer, stainless steel mixing bowl, and individual dessert bowls or goblets

NOTE: *Children should use plastic or table knives for all child steps that require cutting or chopping.*

ADULT & CHILD Crack the eggs on edge of a bowl; with two thumbs in the crack, the child can separate the halves and drop the yolks only into a stainless steel bowl. Freeze whites for future use.

CHILD Help measure the wine and add to the yolks.

ADULT To create a double boiler, place the bowl over a large saucepan filled with just enough water as to not touch the bowl above. Heat the water over medium heat.

ADULT & CHILD Using an electric hand mixer, beat the yolks and wine until well combined.

CHILD Help measure the sugar and salt; add to the yolk mixture.

ADULT & CHILD Beat at high speed for 6 to 8 minutes, or until mixture thickens and mounds.

CHILD Place ¼ cup (36 g) berries in each dessert bowl.

ADULT When zabaglione is thick, remove from heat. Spoon warm sauce over berries and serve immediately. Garnish with a single berry.

PREP TIME	COOK TIME	YIELD
20 minutes	10 minutes	4 servings

PART 5

EXPLORE INTERNATIONAL RECIPE CONCEPTS FOR MORE FLAVOR AND NUTRITION

{DAY 20} Explore the World's Cuisines

WHY ARE VEGETABLES so darned difficult to get past our children? A big part is because American culture never really incorporated fresh vegetables creatively into our cuisine and certainly not with any breadth or depth. Consider some common and popular American recipes: tuna casserole, hamburgers, sloppy joes, chili, meat loaf, hot dogs, fried chicken. The list goes on, but apart from onions, celery, baked beans, cole slaw, and maybe green pepper, tomato, or canned peas on the side, we don't find much in the way of vegetables. Where are the zucchini, kale, eggplant, arugula, cauliflower, and spinach? When you go to a fast-food eatery, do they give you a fabulous side of kale, Brussels sprouts, or cauliflower?

It doesn't matter why things evolved this way. What matters is that as a nation, we're eating too many calories and not getting enough of calories from plant foods—and both are making us fat and harming our health. Yet the irony is that the United States is a pluralistic society of immigrants from many other cultures with rich food traditions that include so many delicious vegetables. We all get Thai and Chinese takeout and find the veggies in these dishes interesting and appealing. But when we prepare meals at home, we unceremoniously plunk our vegetables—unincorporated into the other food and suspect—on the plate next to meat, poultry, or fish. And we serve a whole pile of them! No wonder our kids show little interest in eating them.

MISSION FOR THE DAY

Prepare a new recipe from a culture whose cuisine you have never explored before.

use food to teach kids about other cultures

At home and in our programs, we approach meals for all ages as multicultural adventures. Time and again the result is predictable: an open mind *and* an open mouth! The eater—adult or child—becomes a culinary tourist. Our kids see the world through the prism of food. Each recipe provides a different cultural experience via new ingredients, cooking methods, and the origins of the foods. The best cookbooks dedicated to a singular culture's cooking are successful for these reasons.

Another benefit of our approach is that participants can explore and share their own cultural identities. In our third-grade program, a Vietnamese-American student felt proud of her mother, who volunteered to teach the class how to correctly wrap Vietnamese spring rolls loaded with ginger, carrots, cucumbers, lettuce, mango, and other tasty veggies. The student was the star of the class that day as her classmates happily learned about her culture. As many first- and second-generation Americans become detached from their ethnic backgrounds, exploring and sharing their native foods is an important way for them to reconnect with their cultural identities.

in their own words

If you are skeptical about multicultural recipes, check out some typical comments from our third-grade students:

"I hope to see you in fourth grade because I want to learn more about different cultures. The most interesting culture I studied was Thailand because I never knew that when it rains it makes floods that help rice grow."

"I have really loved cooking class and I have learned a lot. I never really knew that the culture of a country and the climate had so much to do with the food. For example, you told us how people in the Caribbean eat hot food to make them sweat so when the breeze comes they cool off."

"When learning about different cultures I found Asia the most interesting because the food is really different and I could eat healthier there."

"Today I had an Indian feast. We cooked soup with vegetables. I liked the soup and it was fun making the soup."

All our cooking and nutrition education programs are carefully designed to bring a celebratory, festive, and positive spirit to experiential learning with food. This easily translates to the home, where families choose recipes together that embrace colors, smells, textures, and traditions while introducing healthy, plant-based foods. Explore the holidays, rituals, and traditions of other cultures by eating healthy, native dishes. A few online searches will yield information about various cultural traditions—along with lots of tantalizing recipes to try.

We empower children with self-confidence when we help them explore the world around them through the medium of food. The very items that without context seem scary on a plate, such as artichokes or fava beans, become fascinating when presented through the mythology of Italian or Persian culture. The Native American story of the three sisters—corn, bean, and squash—delights children when they hear that in nature these plants "help" each other and have a symbiotic relationship. Folklore gives children a delicious understanding of food and its relationship to nature.

multicultural recipes add spice to everyday meals

Trying out new culinary treats from a wide range of cultures gives your family a welcome break from familiar fare, while also teaching everyone about the associations people around the world attach to food. This list offers a cross section of recipes from the numerous cultures included in this book and promises to give your family a culinary adventure they won't forget:

- ♡ **african and african-american:** Black-Eyed Pea and Collard Soup, Spicy Kenyan Greens
- ♡ **caribbean:** Caribbean Salsa with Snapper, Jamaica Beans and Rice
- ♡ **chinese:** Stir-fry
- ♡ **eastern european:** Date Nut Bars
- ♡ **french:** Fricassee of Vegetables, Zucchini Flan
- ♡ **italian:** Meatless Bolognese, Snap Pea and Mint Pasta, Tuscan Bean Soup, Zabaglione
- ♡ **japanese:** Miso Soup
- ♡ **morocco:** Moroccan Stew
- ♡ **native american:** Spicy Corn Salad, Three Sisters Salad
- ♡ **persian:** Persian Rice with Lentils, Persian New Year Soup
- ♡ **scandinavian:** Barley and Mussels Salad
- ♡ **south american:** Arepas
- ♡ **spain:** Gazpacho, Merche's White Bean and Chorizo Stew
- ♡ **thai:** Chicken and Coconut Milk Soup

But when we prepare meals at home, we unceremoniously plunk our vegetables … on the plate next to meat, poultry, or fish. And we serve a whole pile of them! No wonder our kids show little interest in eating them.

⏱ get started

As you begin your international culinary adventure, follow these guidelines to see how to transform your dinners into a multicultural celebration:

- ♡ Select a food from a culture you would like to explore as a family, using options given in this book.
- ♡ Select a recipe from the culture you have chosen.
- ♡ Invite your children to help you look up historical and nutritional information related to your chosen recipe.
- ♡ Plan a festive evening with the chosen culture as a theme. Download some music, ask your kids to make table decorations, and even plan to watch a movie from that culture after dinner.

jamaican rice and beans

Lynn adopted this recipe from a Jamaican cook in the New York City school system, with whom she worked when she began bringing food education into public schools. This dish is both flavorful and fast to make, so we include it in our curricula.

1 medium onion

2 cloves garlic

⅓ green bell pepper

½ habañero, or Scotch bonnet pepper, or ½ teaspoon hot sauce

1½ tablespoon (25 ml) olive oil

2 cans (15 ounces, or 420 g each) kidney beans

¼ cup (60 ml) coconut milk

2 cups (322 g) cooked rice

½ teaspoon kosher salt

¼ teaspoon freshly ground black pepper

1 large sprig fresh thyme

NOTE: *Children should use plastic or table knives for all child steps that require cutting or chopping.*

ADULT Slice the onion.

CHILD Chop the onion slices into very small pieces.

ADULT Smash the garlic with the flat side of a chef's knife to remove the peel. Slice the garlic.

CHILD Chop the garlic slices into very small pieces.

ADULT Slice the bell pepper.

CHILD Chop the bell pepper slices into very small pieces.

ADULT Slice the habañero thinly, wearing plastic gloves to keep the spicy oils from getting in your eyes if you touch your face.

ADULT Heat the olive oil in a large skillet over medium high heat. Add the onion, garlic, bell pepper, and habañero. Reduce the heat to low and cook vegetables, stirring often, about 10 minutes, or until softened.

ADULT While the veggies are cooking, open the cans of beans and coconut milk.

ADULT & CHILD Rinse the beans in a colander. Measure the coconut milk. Wearing oven mitts to protect hands, add both to the cooked veggies.

ADULT Add the cooked rice, salt, and pepper. Add the entire sprig of fresh thyme. Mix thoroughly and cook on low heat, covered tightly, for 10 to 15 minutes.

PREP TIME	COOK TIME	YIELD
30 minutes	25 minutes	4 to 6 servings

spring pea risotto with herbs

When it comes to what you can do with risotto, this recipe is only the tip of the iceberg. What will be your family's favorite "add in"?

FOR BASIC RISOTTO:

8 cups (1.9 L) chicken broth

1 medium onion

4 tablespoons (57 g) butter, divided

2 tablespoons (30 ml) extra-virgin olive oil

1½ ounces (43 g) Parmigiano-Reggiano cheese

2 cups (421 g) arborio rice

⅓ cup (80 ml) white wine

Kosher salt

OPTIONAL:

Several sprigs fresh basil

Several sprigs fresh flat-leaf Italian parsley

1 bag (10-ounces, or 280 g) frozen peas

NOTE: *Children should use plastic or table knives for all child steps that require cutting or chopping.*

FOR BASIC RISOTTO:

ADULT Heat the chicken broth in a medium saucepan over medium-high heat until boiling. Reduce heat to low and simmer until ready to use.

ADULT Slice the onion.

CHILD Cut the onion slices into a small dice.

ADULT Heat 3 tablespoons (43 g) of the butter and the 2 tablespoons (30 ml) of olive oil in a large stockpot over medium heat.

ADULT Add the onion and cook, stirring occasionally, over low heat, about 10 minutes, or until onions are translucent.

ADULT & CHILD While the onion is cooking, grate the cheese. Set aside.

ADULT & CHILD When the onions are translucent, stir in the rice and continue stirring slowly over medium-high heat until the butter and onion mixture coats each grain of rice and the rice is glistening.

ADULT Stir in the white wine and continue stirring until it is completely absorbed. You are now well into the constant stirring process necessary for good risotto.

ADULT & CHILD Adult demonstrates how to dip a ladle of broth and pour it into the rice. Stir the rice continuously with a long-handled spoon until the broth is absorbed. Child can take turns, repeating this over and over, using the long-handled spoon to stir (hands protected by oven mitts). Continue adding as much broth as necessary until the rice is cooked through but not mushy. The goal is to achieve a creamy consistency, slightly soupy but not watery. You may have broth left over.

ADULT & CHILD Measure and add the remaining 1 tablespoon (14 g) of butter. Stir in grated cheese to taste, just before serving. Season to taste with salt. If you're adding mushrooms, vegetables, or anything else, they should be precooked and stirred in at this stage, *(continued)*

PREP TIME	COOK TIME	YIELD
25 minutes	15 minutes	6 servings

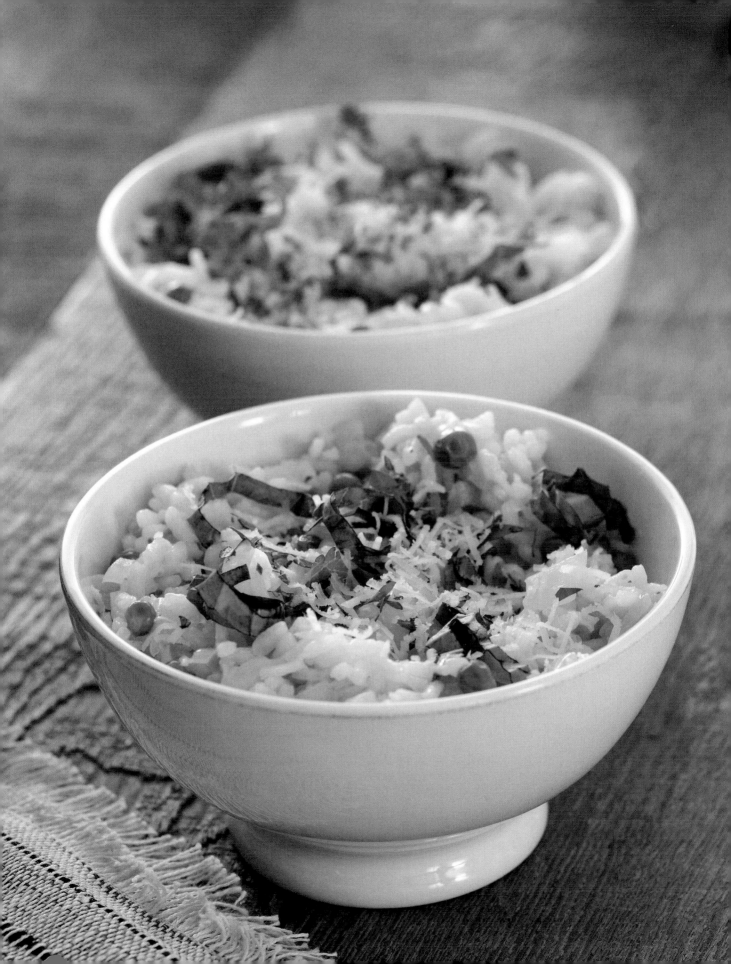

spring pea risotto with herbs *continued*

just before spooning into individual serving bowls. Serve the risotto immediately—risotto does not hold for any length of time.

FOR OPTIONAL INGREDIENTS:
ADULT & CHILD Remove the basil and parsley leaves from their stems and discard the stems. Chop the leaves until you have ½ cup (20 g) of each.

ADULT & CHILD Add the frozen peas to risotto when it is nearly finished. Stir to incorporate; the peas will thaw in a minute or two.

ADULT & CHILD Add the chopped herbs when you add the final tablespoon of butter and the cheese. Mix well.

ADULT Serve immediately.

persian rice with raisins and lentils

Persian cuisine is one of the most sophisticated and healthy, yet undervalued, cuisines we've encountered. This recipe is just one of the delicious plant-based dishes for which this culture is known. Serve with a chunky salad or vegetable soup, and your family will ask for more.

2 cups (370 g) long-grain white basmati rice (you can use brown basmati, but white rice makes the dish prettier because it takes up more of the orange saffron color)

3 tablespoons (45 g) salt, divided

1 cup (192 g) brown lentils

4 tablespoons (57 g) unsalted butter, divided

1 cup (145 g) raisins or currents

1 tablespoon (15 ml) extra virgin olive oil

6 tablespoons (90 ml) water, divided

¼ cup (60 g) plain yogurt, whole or part skim, divided

½ cup (120 ml) very hot water

1½ teaspoons saffron threads

⅔ cup (37 g) slivered almonds

ADDITIONAL COOKING EQUIPMENT:
Mortar and pestle

NOTE: *Children should use plastic or table knives for all child steps that require cutting or chopping.*

ADULT & CHILD In a medium-size bowl, rinse the rice under cool water, changing the water repeatedly until the water runs clear and the excess starch is removed. Place the rice in a bowl and cover with water to 1 inch (2.5 cm) above the rice. Add 2 tablespoons (30 g) of the salt to the water and rice and let sit for one hour.

ADULT & CHILD In another small bowl, rinse the lentils. Place lentils in a bowl and cover with water to 1 inch (2.5 cm) above the lentils and let sit for an hour.

CHILD After the rice has soaked about 40 minutes, help measure 2 tablespoons (28 g) of the butter. Help measure the raisins.

ADULT Melt the 2 tablespoons (28 g) butter in a small skillet over low heat. Add the raisins and cook about 5 minutes, or until softened. Remove from heat and set aside.

ADULT Fill a large stockpot two-thirds full with water. Add remaining 1 tablespoon (15 g) salt and bring to a boil over high heat. Drain the rice and lentils and add to the boiling water. Cook 3 to 5 minutes over medium to high heat. Do not overcook: lentils should still be chewy and not too soft. Drain in a colander.

ADULT & CHILD In the same stockpot, measure and add 1 tablespoon (14 g) of the remaining butter, the olive oil, and 2 tablespoons (30 ml) of the water. Stir together and cook over medium heat until butter is melted. In a small bowl, combine ¾ cup (56 g) rice and lentils with the plain yogurt. Spread over the bottom of the stockpot.

ADULT & CHILD Using a spatula, layer the remaining rice and lentils over the yogurt mixture to form a pyramid shape. *(continued)*

PREP TIME	COOK TIME	YIELD
1 hour 40 minutes 3(includes soaking of the rice and lentils)	90 minutes (combined steps)	4 to 6 servings

persian rice with raisins and lentils *continued*

ADULT In a small saucepan, melt the remaining 1 tablespoon (14 g) of butter and add the ½ cup (120 ml) very hot water. Pour over the rice. Place the lid of the pot in the center of a kitchen towel and pull the ends of the towel up over the knob of the lid. Place the covered lid on the stockpot. Cook over high heat for 20 minutes. Reduce heat to low and steam the rice for 60 minutes (this will form a hard brown crust on the bottom of the pan, known in Farsi as *tadeeg*).

ADULT & CHILD When the rice is nearly cooked, reheat the raisins in the skillet over low heat. Crush the saffron threads in a mortar and pestle or with a wooden spoon in a bowl to form a powder. Add the remaining 4 tablespoons (60 ml) water to the saffron and pour over the raisins. Mix well. Measure and add the slivered almonds to the raisins, and heat together for 2 minutes.

ADULT Spoon half of the rice onto a large platter. Add half the raisin mixture; stir gently to incorporate. Gently mix the balance of the raisin mixture and the remaining rice and lentils in the pot. Stir gently again to mix thoroughly. Layer one spatula full at a time over the rice and lentils on the platter to form a rounded and attractive dome. Leave the tadeeg in the bottom of the pot and cover the pot.

ADULT Place the covered pot in a sink with 1 inch (2.5 cm) of cool water for 5 minutes. Lift the tadeeg, or crunchy rice, from the bottom of the pot. Serve on a separate platter at the same time you serve the rice and lentils. Don't worry if it does not come out in one piece— break up the crunchy bits and serve on top of the rice or on a separate plate.

{DAY 21} Spice Up Your Meals

YOU CAN OFTEN EXPLAIN the difference between an ordinary dish and a fabulous one in a single word: spices. Sure, you can slice an avocado and serve it with a squeeze of lemon as a side dish, but add a dusting of smoked paprika and see what happens. Wow!

get the most from herbs and spices

Traditionally, herbs and spices have been used not only for cooking but for healing purposes as well. Aromatherapy, for instance, taps the pungent aromas of spices and the essential oils in herbs to produce therapeutic effects on the mind, body, and spirit. In fact, herbal medicine remains one of the most prevalent therapies in the world today. For our purposes here, we like to think of herbs and spices as the culinary "ambassadors" of a culture's cuisine.

Maybe you don't know much about Morocco, but one bite of our Morrocan Vegetable Stew with Butternut Squash will pique your curiosity. In our

use less salt, get more flavor

Lynn never puts a salt shaker on the table, and no one asks for it, because she salts food at the end of the cooking process to enhance natural flavors and bring the many flavors into balance and harmony. She frequently uses sea salt for taste and texture rather than table or kosher salt—a small sprinkle brings out delicious flavors.

MISSION FOR THE DAY

Select a spice or herb that's new to you and use it in a recipe.

curricula, children and adults alike are amazed at how different herbs and spices transform the flavor of familiar vegetables or recipes into something astonishingly different. Our second-grade lesson from our "Look Who's Cooking" program starts with an exploration of exotic African spices and aromas to draw the children in. Our "Teen Battle Chefs" prefer to make veggie tacos (see recipe in this chapter) that use tempeh instead of ground meat. Why? Because the tempeh absorbs the incredible flavor of chipotle and ancho chili powders more than ground beef does. When you use spices and fresh herbs in your recipes, you add so much flavor you'll need much less salt.

use more fresh herbs, gain more flavor

Herbs are a fixture in Lynn's kitchen. Her favorites grow only a few steps away from her kitchen so she can cut a few strands each day to add to summer recipes. She often snips as many different types as she has growing and chops, then sprinkles them on flatbread slathered with ricotta cheese. She adds a drizzle of olive oil and a few grains of salt on top—voilà!—an ultrasimple, whole-food snack. She rarely uses dried herbs, especially basil or dill, because these herbs are available fresh all year round. Some

10 best ideas for adding exotic flavors to your meals

region	typical spices used	typical herbs used
northern europe	Anise, caraway, cardamom, cinnamon, cloves, coriander seed, fennel, juniper, nutmeg, pepper, powdered ginger, vanilla	Bay leaf, chervil, chives, dill, parsley, tarragon, thyme,
southern europe	Anise, cayenne pepper, coriander seed, cumin, fennel, pepper, red pepper flakes, saffron	Basil, lavender, marjoram, oregano, parsley, rosemary, sage, savory, thyme
eastern europe	Allspice, angelica, caraway, celery seed, cinnamon, cloves, coriander seed, juniper, mustard seed, paprika (spicy and mild), poppy seed, vanilla	bay leaf, chives, dill, horseradish, marjoram, mint, parsley
africa	Allspice, black pepper, cayenne pepper, cinnamon, cloves, ginger, nutmeg, saffron, sesame, tamarind, vanilla	Cilantro, parsley
middle east	Angelica, fresh ginger, orange water, rosewater, saffron, sesame, sumac, turmeric, za'atar (spice mix)	Dill, mint, parsley
southeast asia	Cardamom, chilies, cinnamon, coconut, coriander seed, curry leaf, curry powder, ginger, mace, nutmeg, star anise, tamarind, wasabi	Basil, bay leaf, cilantro, galangal, lemongrass, lime leaves, mint
india	Black mustard seed, cardamom, cinnamon, garamasala (spice blend), ginger, rosewater, tamarind, turmeric	Cilantro, lemongrass, mint
caribbean	Annatto seeds, cayenne pepper, chilies, coconut, cumin, vanilla, tamarind	Cilantro, epazote, parsley
mexico and central america	Annatto seeds, chili powders, chilies, cinnamon, clove, coconut, cumin, vanilla	Cilantro, epazote, oregano, parsley, thyme
south america	Annatto seeds, chilies	Cilantro, oregano, thyme

dried herbs, such as rosemary, oregano, and sage, are more useful in cooking than other herbs because their flavors remain more pungent in the dried state.

One of our introductory tactics is to prepare cooked fresh carrots in a bit of butter and divide them into several bowls, adding a different freshly chopped herb to each bowl. Again, children and adults are surprised at the burst of flavor and new personalities that boring old carrots take on when dusted with fragrant dill, basil, thyme, mint, or cilantro. Try this exercise with your favorite vegetable or recipe and discover your preference.

Tips for Using Spices
The following suggestions will help you get the most benefits from your spices:

♡ Store spices tightly sealed in glass jars or tins; replace every four to five years, as they lose flavor over time.
♡ Buy whole spices—especially nutmeg, cumin, coriander, mustard seed, fennel, anise, caraway, cloves, and allspice—and using a small mortar and pestle or microplane grater, grind them at home for more flavor.
♡ When possible, buy spices at ethnic grocery stores to get the best prices and flavor.

Tips for Using Fresh Herbs

♡ Put fresh herbs in the fridge to extend their potency. Rinse in water, wrap in a damp paper towel, and store in a plastic bag or container.
♡ Add more than the recipe calls for to increase the "wow" factor.
♡ Put fresh herbs in dishes where you might not ordinarily use them. Experiment with adding them to salads, eggs, toast and cheese, and sauces—get creative.

In our curricula, children and adults alike are amazed at how different herbs and spices transform the flavor of familiar vegetables or recipes into something astonishingly different.

get started

Have you ever visited a spice store? We recommend it. The fresh scents plus the opportunity to explore, sample, and pick up tips is well worth a couple hours of your time. A few national chains and ethnic stores sell spices. If you can't find what you want at a store near you, try shopping online—it's less fun, but you'll find lots of options available. Here are some tips to get you started:

♡ Keep your favorite spices on hand in your pantry.
♡ Using a window box, grow as many types of herbs as you think you'll need. Add more as your culinary repertoire expands.
♡ Experiment with using new herbs and spices in the dishes you prepare for your family. Get feedback from family members. Which flavors do they like?

veggie tacos

As you layer the delectable tempeh chili on the grilled eggplant slices, consider putting arugula or other baby greens or sprouts on top with a slice of avocado—delicious!

2 medium eggplants

4 tablespoons (60 ml) olive oil, divided

Sea salt

1 large onion

2 large cloves garlic

1 pound (455 g) tempeh

2 tablespoons (15 g) ancho chili powder

1 tablespoon (7.5 g) chipotle chili powder

1 can (15 ounces, or 420 g) whole tomatoes

Freshly ground black pepper

1 bunch cilantro

2 ripe avocados

4 cups (220 g) mesclun greens or baby mustard greens

NOTE: *Children should use plastic or table knives for all child steps that require cutting or chopping.*

ADULT & CHILD Slice the eggplants thinly into at least 12 slices.

CHILD Brush the eggplant with thin layer of olive oil and salt lightly.

ADULT Slice the onion. Smash garlic with the flat side of a chef's knife to remove the peel and slice.

CHILD Chop the onion and garlic into very small pieces.

ADULT Heat a large skillet, and add 3 tablespoons (45 ml) of the oil.

ADULT & CHILD Add the onion and garlic. Cook over low heat about 7 minutes, or until translucent (child using oven mitts to protect hands).

ADULT & CHILD Crumble the tempeh and add to the onion mixture. Cook for 2 minutes, mixing well.

ADULT & CHILD Measure and add the ancho and chipotle chili powders to the tempeh.

ADULT Open the can of tomatoes.

ADULT & CHILD Squeeze each tomato to crush it and add it and its juice to the tempeh mixture. Mix well and season to taste with salt and pepper. Cook 5 minutes more.

ADULT While the tempeh is cooking, set oven to low broil, and broil eggplant slices until browned (or cook on a grill pan or outdoor grill until softened).

CHILD Help remove all the cilantro leaves from the stems and discard the stems. Chop the leaves until you have about ½ cup (8 g). Stir the cilantro into the tempeh mixture, and remove from the heat.

CHILD Peel and then slice each avocado into 12 slices.

ADULT & CHILD To serve, place 2 broiled eggplant slices on each plate. Spoon some tempeh, a slice of avocado, and a few pieces of baby greens onto each taco. Top with cilantro.

PREP TIME	COOK TIME	YIELD
20 minutes	15 minutes	6 servings

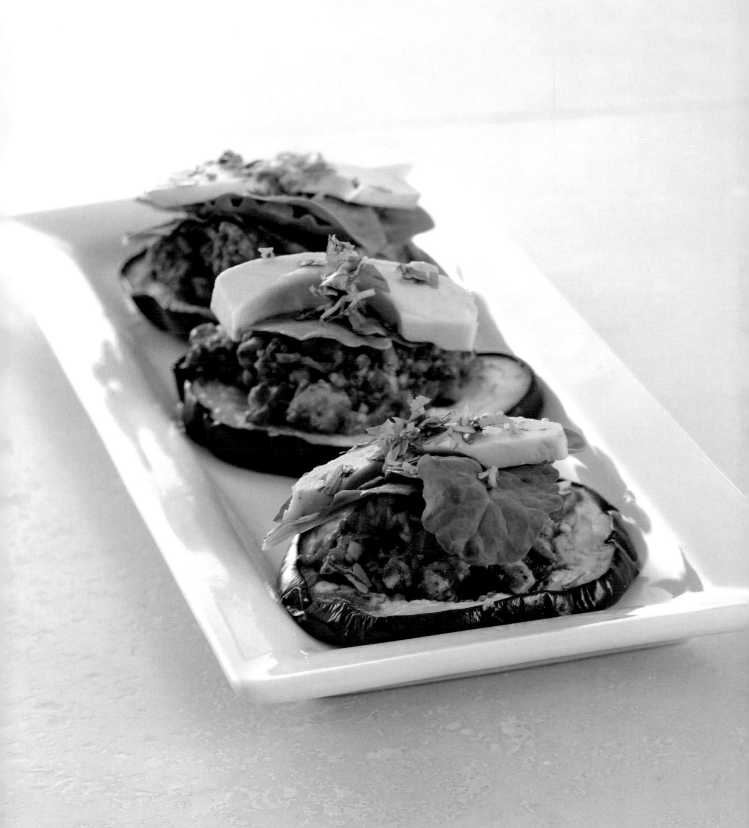

moroccan vegetable stew

The balance of flavors and hint of spice in this recipe make it aromatic and amazingly satisfying, whether or not you add the chicken. Served over whole wheat couscous, it's a filling and delicious meal.

1 medium sweet potato or yam

1 onion

2 tablespoons (30 ml) olive oil

½ pound (225 g) green beans

2 carrots

1 zucchini or other summer squash

2 tablespoons (14 g) paprika

1 teaspoon ground cinnamon

⅛ teaspoon ground nutmeg

½ teaspoon ground cumin

½ teaspoon saffron threads

1 can (28 ounces, or 794 g) whole tomatoes

1 cup (100 g) peas or sliced snap peas

¼ cup (35 g) raisins (optional)

1 can (15 ounces, or 420 g) chickpeas, drained

12 ounces (340 g) diced cooked chicken (optional)

Kosher salt and freshly ground pepper

1½ cups (236 g) whole wheat couscous or cooked brown rice, quinoa, or bulgar

NOTE: *Children should use plastic or table knives for all child steps that require cutting or chopping.*

FOR THE STEW:

CHILD Peel the sweet potato.

ADULT Cube the sweet potato and place in medium saucepan. Cover with water and cook over medium heat until just tender.

ADULT Peel and slice the onion.

CHILD Help chop the onion slices.

ADULT Heat the olive oil in a large stockpot over medium heat. Add the chopped onions, and reduce heat to low. Cook for 5 to 10 minutes, or until softened.

CHILD Trim the green beans. Slice the beans into bite-size pieces.

ADULT Slice the carrots and zucchini. Before the potatoes are completely cooked, add the carrots and beans to the saucepan with the potatoes and blanch for 3 minutes.

CHILD Measure the paprika, cinnamon, nutmeg, cumin, and saffron and add to the onion. Add the tomatoes, squeezing each by hand to break into bite-size pieces, adding the remaining liquid at the end. Add the peas and zucchini. Stir to combine and cook 10 more minutes.

ADULT Drain the boiled vegetables and add to the tomato mixture. Stir in raisins and chickpeas. Add chicken. Cook 5 more minutes, or until all ingredients are evenly heated.

ADULT Season to taste with salt and pepper.

FOR THE COUSCOUS:

ADULT While the vegetables are cooking, bring 3 cups (710 ml) of water to a boil in a medium saucepan with a lid.

ADULT Add the couscous to the boiling water, stir once, and cover with the lid; turn off the heat. Let stand 10 minutes.

ADULT When you are ready to serve, uncover the couscous and fluff with a wooden spoon. Serve the vegetable stew over the couscous.

PREP TIME	COOK TIME	YIELD
15 minutes	30 to 40 minutes	4 to 6 servings

{DAY 22} Explore Asian Flavors

KIDS GENERALLY LIKE CHINESE TAKEOUT. What's not to like? There's lots of flavor, no one food dominates the plate, plus most Chinese dishes are colorful and very easy to eat. No need for Mom or Dad to cut up anything since each dish comes in bite-size pieces.

Asian cuisine is inherently healthy and balanced. Each dish uses a variety of colorful vegetables and a grain, and uses less meat as it often includes plant proteins such as beans, tofu, and legumes. Hence they're less expensive to make. The many variations make meals interesting and appealing to your family. By preparing these dishes yourself, you can choose the freshest quality ingredients and avoid the additives that many Asian take-out restaurants use.

Most of us would not be afraid to make the most common Asian dish, a stir-fry—a simple dish with veggies and meat. Now that your sous chefs are comfortable in the kitchen, they can help you prep—and the cooking part takes only minutes.

build delicious flavor into an asian stir-fry

Here is the basic "architecture" for preparing a stir-fry:

1. Heat vegetable oil in a hot wok and infuse aromatics (garlic, ginger, etc.) into the oil.
2. Add the ingredients that will take the longest to cook (meat or dense vegetables, such as cauliflower or broccoli).
3. Add the ingredients that will take the least amount of time to cook (delicate veggies that

> **MISSION FOR THE DAY**
>
> Create a stir-fry from the ingredients in your pantry, fresh seasonal produce, and our basic stir-fry recipe concept.

cook quickly, such as string beans, leafy greens, snap peas).
4. Add the liquid seasonings (e.g., soy or fish sauce) and finishing touches (garnishes, herbs).

Now, we're sure that if you taste a Cantonese stir-fry side by side with a Thai version containing many of the same ingredients, such as beef or chicken and similar vegetables, you will notice they taste entirely different. That's because each culture has a different flavor profile and approach. Refer to the chart on page 150 to see the key ingredients that set these culinary traditions apart.

After that you see the distinctions among ingredients, it's easy to understand how the same type of dish can be distinctly Chinese or Thai. With just the following bit of knowledge, you can take any basic Chinese or Thai stir-fry and make your own.

Chinese Stir-Fry Basics

For a Chinese dish, you will generally be infusing the oil with garlic and then possibly chilies or ginger or some other aromatic. After the aromatics have had a chance to penetrate the oil, you begin adding the meat and then vegetables. If you are adding seafood, add it at the end because it cooks so quickly. In

ingredients that will help unlock your inner asian chef		
	chinese	thai/vietnamese
fat	Peanut or canola oil	Peanut or canola oil
sweet	Sugar	Coconut milk, palm sugar, sweet soy, tamarind
salt	Oyster sauce, sesame oil, soy sauce	Fish sauce, Thai oyster sauce
sour	Rice vinegar	Limes, pickled garlic, pickled radish, tamarind
aromatics	Garlic, ginger, onion, scallions	Galangal, garlic, ginger, kafir limes, lemongrass, shallots
chiles	Sichuan chiles, chile sauce and paste	Long hot chiles (you can substitute jalapeño), tiny fresh "bird" chiles, siracha (chile sauce)
herbs	Coriander seed, chives	Cilantro and cilantro root, holy or Thai basil (you can substitute regular Italian basil), mint
rice	Short-grain rice	Jasmine rice

this way, everything is nearly cooked to perfection and veggies are still crunchy. Before serving, add the finishing touch of seasonings.

Thai Stir-Fry Basics

In a Thai version, you generally pound some chilies and shallots and maybe coriander or lemongrass in a mortar and pestle, then infuse the oil with that. Next you cook the meat and add the vegetables. When the cooking is nearly done, add fish sauce, fresh herbs, and limes. You may even add some palm sugar to create more harmony among the sweet, salty, bitter, and spicy flavors.

asian soups are quick to make and full of flavor

Asian soups are some of the quickest, most flavorful meals you can prepare. Traditionally, these recipes are composed of pretty specific veggies. But we take license with tradition and serve them brimming with colorful seasonal vegetables. The flavors could

not be more different, but both are tasty crowd pleasers. The miso soup has been a staple in our school programs for nearly fifteen years. Another plus—you can have dinner ready in fifteen minutes!

Our soup recipes can also be modified to please your family's palates. We've indicated with an asterisk the ingredients that can be changed.

get started

Your kids will love helping you prepare these colorful and flavorful dishes. After you've tried the basic recipes, experiment with your own variations. Here are some ideas to help you get started:

- ♡ Choose a stir-fry and a soup concept to try over the next week.
- ♡ Purchase Asian pantry staples listed earlier in this chapter.
- ♡ Have fun swapping out some ingredients for variety.

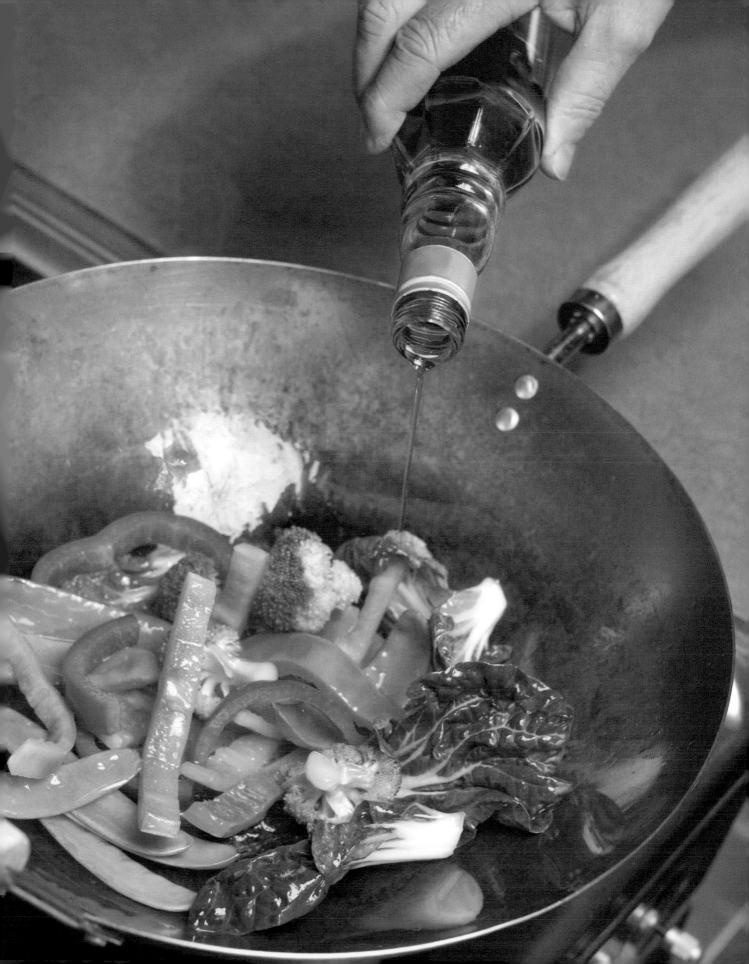

miso soup with shrimp

When Mercedes lived in Japan, the comforting flavor of miso soup won her over to Japanese food. Once you make the broth, experiment with adding veggies. The fermented soy will support the friendly bacteria in your digestive system.

4 cups (946 ml) canned fish broth, or use bouillon cubes

4 tablespoons (64 g) miso paste

4 ounces (115 g) shiitake mushrooms*

4 ounces (115 g) firm tofu*

1 dozen medium shrimp*

4 scallions

NOTE: *Children should use plastic or table knives for all child steps that require cutting or chopping.*

ADULT Heat the fish broth in a medium saucepan over medium heat until it comes to a simmer. Place the miso paste in a small bowl.

ADULT & CHILD Measure 3 tablespoons (45 ml) of the heated broth and add it to the miso paste. Whisk with a small wire whisk to dissolve the miso. When it is a smooth consistency, adult blends the miso back into the saucepan of broth and mixes well. Continue simmering the broth.

CHILD Remove the stems from the mushrooms and discard.

CHILD Slice the mushroom caps into 3 or 4 slices each.

CHILD Cut the tofu into small cubes.

CHILD Peel the shrimp.

CHILD Slice the scallions.

ADULT Add the shiitake and tofu to the simmering miso broth. Cook 3 minutes.

ADULT & CHILD Add the shelled shrimp and cook about 4 minutes, or until the shrimp are completely pink. Do not overcook.

ADULT & CHILD Add the sliced scallions and mix well. Simmer 2 minutes more.

ADULT Ladle soup into bowls.

PREP TIME	COOK TIME	YIELD
20 minutes	10 minutes	4 servings

thai chicken and coconut milk soup

When Lynn prepares this soup, her family and friends can't get enough of it. We make it pretty spicy, so it really clears out the sinuses—it's especially welcome on a cold day.

2 cups (475 ml) chicken broth

1 can (13 or 15 ounces, or 364 or 420 g) coconut milk (full fat, not "lite")

1 large shallot

1 long lemongrass

5 to 6 (minimum) tiny Thai chile peppers, or 1 or 2 jalapeños

3 to 4 cilantro roots

3 boneless chicken thighs

⅓ pound (152 g) each of at least 3 types of colorful vegetables (yellow pepper, mushrooms, snap peas, Thai or other eggplants, cabbage)ᴬ

2-inch (5-cm) piece frozen galangal (optional)

1 to 2 tablespoons (15 to 30 ml) fish sauce (for salt)

Juice of 2 limes

1 to 3 teaspoons (4 to 12 g) sugar

3 to 4 sprigs Thai (or Italian) basil

3 to 4 sprigs mint

ADDITIONAL COOKING EQUIPMENT:
Mortar and pestle

NOTE: *Children should use plastic or table knives for all child steps that require cutting or chopping.*

ADULT Bring the broth and coconut milk to a boil in a medium saucepan over medium heat.

ADULT Slice the shallot, lemongrass, chilies, and cilantro roots.

ADULT & CHILD Using a mortar and pestle, bruise and crush the sliced ingredients to release their flavor and oils.

ADULT & CHILD Add to the boiling liquid and let simmer 5 minutes.

ADULT Meanwhile, cut the chicken into bite-size pieces and add to the broth. Cook 4 to 6 minutes, or until chicken is almost cooked through.

ADULT Cut the colorful vegetables into slices.

CHILD Help cut the vegetable slices into bite-size pieces. Add to the broth.

ADULT Slice the galangal, if using, and add to broth.

ADULT & CHILD Using "tasting" spoons, add fish sauce, lime juice, and sugar a little at a time and taste until a satisfying balance is achieved.

CHILD Remove leaves from the basil and mint stems and chop. Add a handful to each bowl before the hot soup is ladled in.

ADULT Serve hot with more lime and chilies available for people who desire more heat.

PREP TIME	COOK TIME	YIELD
20 minutes	15 minutes	4 servings

chinese rainbow stir-fry

Here we provide a base for an infinite variety of future meals—play with different seafood, fish, meat, and veggies, focusing on what's in season.

1 large head broccoli

2 cloves garlic

1 piece ginger 3 inches (7.5 cm) long

½ cup (120 ml) peanut oil

1 pound (455 g) boneless chicken breast*

1 medium red bell pepper*

1 small yellow squash*

¼ cup (60 ml) soy sauce

¼ cup (60 ml) oyster sauce

1 tablespoon (8 g) toasted sesame seeds

4 cups (640 g) cooked brown rice

ADDITIONAL COOKING EQUIPMENT:
Wok (optional)

NOTE: *Children should use plastic or table knives for all child steps that require cutting or chopping.*

tip

If you can't find toasted seeds, toast them yourself:

- Heat a dry skillet over medium heat.
- Add the sesame seeds and stir constantly.
- Cook 5 minutes, or until they become evenly browned.

CHILD Cut the broccoli into bite-size flowerets.

ADULT & CHILD Adult smashes the garlic with the flat side of a chef's knife to remove peel and slices. Child minces the garlic finely.

CHILD Peel the ginger.

ADULT Slice the ginger for child to mince finely.

ADULT Heat the peanut oil in a wok or large nonstick skillet over high heat.

ADULT Slice the chicken into thin slices. Cut the slices into 1½-inch (2.5 cm)-long pieces.

ADULT Add the garlic and ginger to the hot oil and stir fry 2 minutes, stirring constantly.

ADULT Add the meat to the oil and stir fry 3 minutes, stirring constantly.

ADULT Slice the bell pepper (seeds and membrane removed) and squash into ½-inch (13 mm) strips.

CHILD Cut the red bell pepper strips into smaller, bite-size pieces. Cut the squash into semi-circles. Slice the scallions thinly.

ADULT Add the broccoli to the wok and stir fry for 2 minutes. Continue to supervise cutting of remaining vegetables.

ADULT & CHILD Add the bell pepper, yellow squash, and scallions, stirring constantly.

ADULT & CHILD Measure and add the soy and oyster sauces.

ADULT Taste seasoning, adding more soy or oyster sauce as needed. Remove from heat and stir in toasted sesame seeds. Serve over rice.

PREP TIME	COOK TIME	YIELD
25 minutes	15 minutes	4 to 6 servings

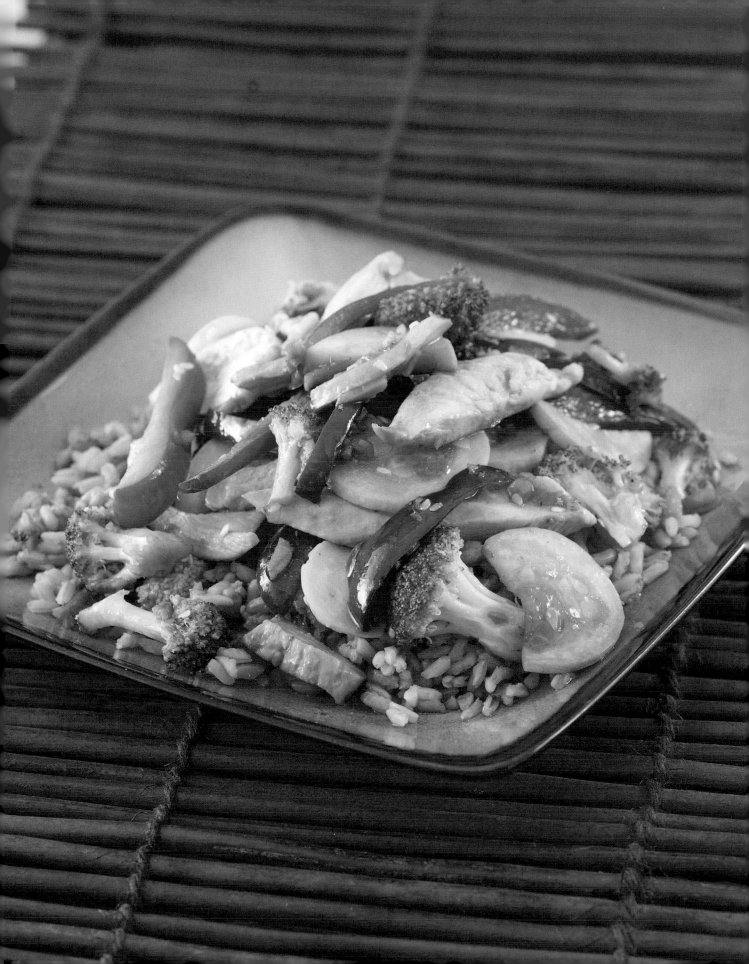

thai chili and basil stir-fry

The classic Thai combination of hot chilies, garlic, and basil complements meat, fish, and chicken. Like Chinese stir-fry, you can invent endless variations.

5 to 6 small Thai chilies, or 2 jalapeños

4 cloves garlic

2 tablespoons (30 ml) canola oil

1 shallot

1 tablespoons (13 g) sugar

2 tablespoons (30 ml) fish sauce

1 tablespoon (15 ml) sweet or regular soy sauce

½ tablespoon (8 ml) oyster sauce

1 cup (100 g) green beans*

1¼ pound (567 g) lean ground beef*

4 fresh or frozen kaffir lime leaves, shredded (optional)*

¾ cup (175 ml) chicken broth

10 holy basil leaves or regular basil

3 scallions

4 cups (640 g) cooked Thai jasmine or brown rice

ADDITIONAL COOKING EQUIPMENT:
Wok (optional)

NOTE: *Children should use plastic or table knives for all child steps that require cutting or chopping.*

ADULT Slice the hot chilies. Smash the garlic with the flat side of a chef's knife to remove peel and slice thinly.

ADULT Heat a wok or large nonstick skillet and add oil. Stir-fry the chilies and garlic for 2 minutes.

ADULT & CHILD Slice the shallot. Add to the stir-fry and cook for 2 minutes.

ADULT & CHILD Measure and add the sugar, fish sauce, soy sauce, and oyster sauce. Trim and cut the green beans in half. Add to the stir-fry.

ADULT Add the ground beef and brown as you break it up with a wooden spoon.

ADULT Add lime leaves and the chicken broth. Stir-fry another 5 to 8 minutes. Taste and adjust seasonings (fish, soy and oyster sauces) to taste. Add basil and stir-fry until just wilted. Serve with sliced scallion garnish and jasmine rice.

PREP TIME	**COOK TIME**	**YIELD**
15 minutes	15 minutes	4 servings

{DAY 23} Eat Like a Roman

ONE OF THE MOST TALENTED and famous Northern Italian chefs (in his day) was once Lynn's client. She learned so much about flavor and Italian cooking from Andreas Hellrigl, the chef of the grand New York City restaurant Palio in the 1980s and 1990s. What were his secrets? Employing simplicity, pure ingredients, and careful combination, and letting the ingredients speak for themselves.

Italian cuisine is arguably the ultimate comfort food of the Mediterranean. As Lynn endeavored to raise her sons with good nutrition and plenty of quality family time, she often turned to Italian cuisine because her children never complained when she served it. She could add the dreaded "green things" to the family meal, but as long as the pasta or risotto or gnocchi were present on their plates—*silenzio!*

Even today when Lynn needs to produce a meal quickly, she knows the carefully planned Italian staples in her pantry, fridge, and freezer will save the day. The chart of basics on page 158 provide multiple menu possibilities. By keeping these staples on hand, she can whip up a meal in about as long as it takes to cook dry pasta. You can, too.

italian snacks and hors d'oeuvres are quick and easy to make

Whether it's a traditional antipasti of olives, peppers, Italian cheese, and salami, or the more elegant melon with prosciutto, or prosciutto wound around breadsticks with pickled caper berries and olives, the Italians have some of the most satisfying and fridge-friendly hors d'oeuvres. Here are some other quick-and-easy tidbits for snacks and entertaining that are always a hit with kids and adults alike.

Crostini
These little garlic toasts with toppings are some of Lynn's family's favorites. Consider using the following toppings:

- ♡ fresh tomato, basil, garlic, and olive oil combined until saucy
- ♡ caramelized red onions
- ♡ green or black olive spread
- ♡ artichoke spread
- ♡ pesto with fresh mozzarella
- ♡ chicken liver pâté
- ♡ white beans and garlic mashed with extra-virgin olive oil

> **MISSION FOR THE DAY**
>
> Invent your own Italian pasta dish.

157

best italian staples to keep on hand for quick meals		
pantry	fridge	freezer
Quality extra-virgin olive oil	Fresh garlic	Ravioli
Quality balsamic vinegar (no additives)	Greens (spinach, arugula, kale, chard)	Fettuccini
Basil pesto	Parmigiano-Reggiano or grana padano cheese	Basil puree in ice cube trays
Walnut sauce	Pancetta	Italian sausage (mild)
Sun-dried tomato pesto	Broccoli rabe, fennel	Italian sausage (hot)
Pine nuts	Onions or shallots	Clams
Red pepper flakes	Ricotta cheese	Shrimp or langoustine
Canned crushed tomatoes	Herbs	Fresh gnocchi
2 to 3 types small pasta and long pasta	Olives	
Bread crumbs	Heavy cream	
Flat bread	Scallions	
Tapenade		
Red wine vinegar		

Flatbread
Spread flatbread with ricotta cheese and finish with assorted toppings. Here are some family favorites from Lynn's kitchen:

- ♡ fresh-snipped sage, rosemary, basil, and parsley, drizzled with extra-virgin olive oil and a sprinkle of sea salt
- ♡ fresh, sweet cherry tomatoes with basil and some quality olive oil and sea salt
- ♡ sliced figs, rosemary, and prosciutto

special italian jar sauces save time and fuss
No, we don't mean the standard, supermarket-type tomato sauces that come in a jar—we're going to teach you how to make your own savory sauce in almost no time at all (see right). The jar sauces we are zeroing in on here are not tomato sauces and do not even need to be heated. These special Italian sauces will arm you with diverse pasta flavoring options. They will last a long time in your fridge or pantry and can be used as needed in emergencies or on days when you want the comfort of a lovely pasta or ravioli without the fuss.

fabulous italian sauces for your pantry	
basil pesto	Add to any type or shape pasta, including ravioli. Add toasted pine nuts for crunch, cherry tomatoes in season, or parboiled veggies, such as snap peas, zucchini, or yellow squash.
sun-dried tomato pesto	Use similarly to the basil pesto. It tastes particularly delicious with cheese or goat cheese ravioli. Add sliced and browned Italian sausage—instant dinner.
walnut sauce	Use similarly to the pestos, but because of its earthy flavor, pair it with meat and other filled pastas, such as tortellini filled with prosciutto. It's also wonderful with sautéed mushrooms and long pasta.
black olive tapenade	Serve over spaghetti or linguine, add crushed cherry tomatoes and basil. Great side dish with chicken tenders coated in olive oil and bread crumbs and sautéed.

get started

Expand your ideas about pasta dishes, and venture beyond the familiar tomato sauce. By stocking your pantry with even a few of the Italian staples we recommend, you can turn out quick cuisine that pleases everyone. Here are some ideas to get you started:

- ♡ Stock basic Italian pantry and fridge staples, based on the suggestions listed in the chart. You don't need everything, but some from each list will be lifesavers.
- ♡ Choose one recipe in this chapter to try.
- ♡ Go to the farmers' market and select the most inspiring produce; use it in your chosen recipe.

quick marinara sauce

Every Italian family has a tomato sauce recipe they swear by. But Lynn's Italian chef client had an amazing strategy for making a quick tomato sauce base, to which he could add meat or seafood, seasonal veggies, capers, and olives. Each option takes the base sauce in a new flavor direction. Here's the secret sauce—you'll love it!

2 cloves very fresh garlic

1 small onion

3 tablespoons (45 ml) extra-virgin olive oil

Pinch of red pepper flakes

1 can (28 ounces, or 794 g) crushed tomatoes

NOTE: *Children should use plastic or table knives for all child steps that require cutting or chopping.*

ADULT Smash the garlic cloves with the flat end of a chef's knife to remove peel. Slice the garlic.

CHILD Chop the garlic slices finely.

ADULT Slice the onion.

CHILD Chop the onion slices finely.

ADULT Heat the olive oil in a medium skillet over medium-high heat. Add the garlic, onions, and red pepper flakes. Reduce heat to medium-low and cook 5 minutes, or until garlic is golden.

ADULT Add the crushed tomatoes, stirring to incorporate all the garlic and hot pepper. Increase heat to medium and bring sauce to a simmer. Continue simmering 5 to 8 minutes more.

PREP TIME	COOK TIME	YIELD
10 minutes	10 minutes	3 to 4 cups (750 to 1000 g)

spring farfalle with asparagus

This is a delightful recipe to make in spring and summer—you can swap out the asparagus for spinach, broccoli rabe, Swiss chard. Adjust cooking time based on the vegetable you use. You may also want to change the herbs to basil or sage, depending on what vegetable or greens you choose.

1 teaspoon salt

1 pound (455 g) asparagus

8 ounces (225 g) whole wheat penne or farfalle

2 cloves garlic

3 tablespoons (45 ml) extra-virgin olive oil

1 teaspoon red pepper flakes

3 tablespoons (12 g) Italian parsley

3 tablespoons (27 g) toasted pine nuts

Parmigiano-Reggiano cheese for grating

Salt and freshly ground black pepper

NOTE: *Children should use plastic or table knives for all child steps that require cutting or chopping.*

ADULT Bring a large saucepan of water to boil for the pasta. Add a teaspoon of salt and bring back to a boil.

ADULT & CHILD While the water for pasta is heating, cut the asparagus lengthwise, and then into 1-inch (2.5 cm) pieces.

ADULT Add the pasta to the boiling water and cook for 7 minutes.

ADULT Smash the garlic with the flat end of a chef's knife to remove the peel, and slice.

CHILD Chop the garlic.

ADULT Heat a large skillet over medium heat. Add the olive oil, garlic, and red pepper flakes. Sauté until garlic is browned; lower heat if they are browning too quickly and risk burning. After pasta has cooked for 7 minutes, add the asparagus to the pasta. Cook for 2 minutes.

CHILD While the pasta and asparagus are cooking together, help chop the parsley.

ADULT Meanwhile add parsley and a ladle of pasta water to the oil and garlic. Add toasted pine nuts and simmer for 2 minutes.

ADULT With a sieve, scoop the pasta and asparagus, allowing the water to drain back into the saucepan, and transfer to the skillet. Add additional pasta water to make the mixture saucy.

CHILD Grate the cheese to sprinkle over each serving.

ADULT Cook until pasta is al dente or still slightly chewy. Serve with the grated cheese, and season to taste with salt and freshly ground pepper.

PREP TIME	COOK TIME	YIELD
10 minutes	20 minutes	4 servings

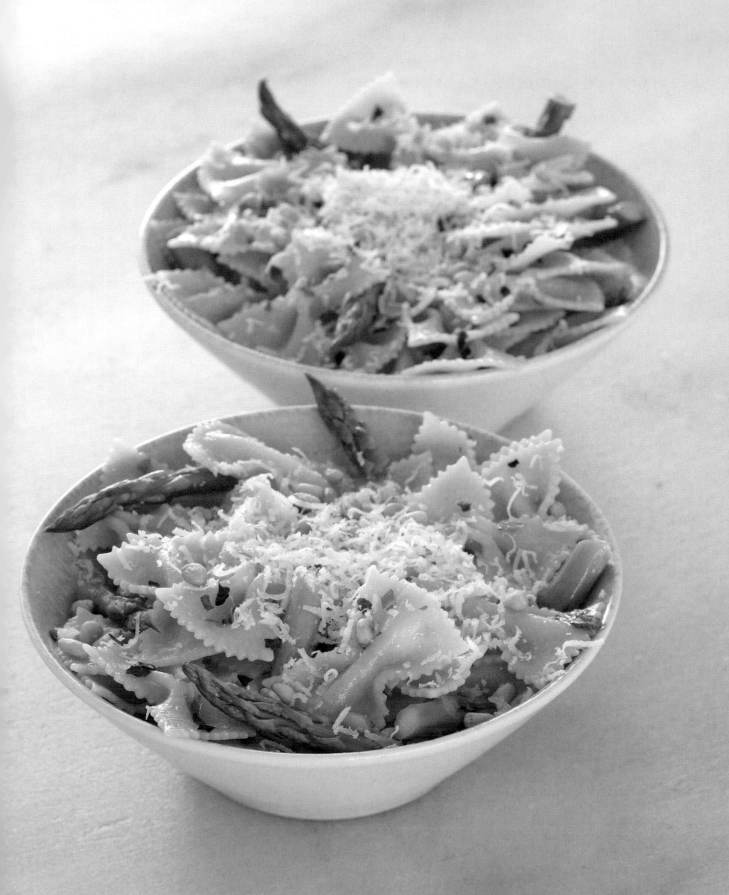

jimmy's favorite macaroni

One of the first meals Lynn's children cooked for themselves is "Jimmy's Favorite Macaroni," named after her good friend Jimmy Ienner, Jr. Jimmy is Italian and grew up on macaroni, as his family calls all pasta. His mother devised this recipe, which is hugely popular with kids and adults who appreciate its wholesome simplicity. The ricotta cheese not only adds flavor and texture but also protein and calcium to this meal.

1 pound (455 g) spaghetti

1 jar (28 ounces, or 794 g) marinara sauce

1⅓ cups (335 g) ricotta cheese (part skim is fine), divided

NOTE: *Children should use plastic or table knives for all child steps that require cutting or chopping.*

tip

To add some veggies, grate your favorite root vegetable on top of the ricotta before you add the pasta and sauce.

ADULT Bring a large saucepan of water to boil. Add the pasta and cook until al dente, or still slightly chewy.

ADULT Heat the marinara sauce in a small saucepan over medium heat until hot enough to serve.

CHILD Help measure and spread ⅓ cup (85 g) of the ricotta cheese in a thin layer on each of 4 plates.

ADULT Drain the pasta and divide evenly among each plate, placing it over the cheese to melt it.

ADULT & CHILD After about 2 minutes, spoon the warm sauce over pasta and serve.

PREP TIME	COOK TIME	YIELD
5 minutes	5 minutes	4 servings

PART 6

TIME-SAVING STRATEGIES FOR SUPER MEALS

{DAY 24} Tap Time-Saving Techniques

IF YOU ARE LIKE A LOT OF PARENTS, you don't want to take a shortcut on quality, but would love to spend less time on kitchen duties. In this chapter, we'll summarize some techniques that will help you prepare meals more quickly and efficiently.

Because this book is about cooking from scratch with fresh ingredients, you can't avoid meal planning and shopping. On Days 4 through 6, we offer a window into efficiency with our strategies for menu planning and shopping by season and concepts. On Days 11 through 12, we provide tips for cooking smarter and bringing your children into the kitchen to help you. Now we'll build on previous guidance.

convenient cooking doesn't mean serving convenience foods

We're going to make a distinction here between convenient and convenience. Busy parents want to learn ways to make planning and preparing meals more convenient. But our goal is to provide healthy strategies, and that means we eschew most convenience food products that are highly processed.

more time-saving tips to make meals easier

♡ Pay your babysitter for extra time each week to help with some of the shopping and vegetable prepping; or do major cooking when the cleaning person is there to help you. Of course, if you have teens this is a great job for them.

MISSION
FOR THE DAY
———
Use one technique from this chapter to save time.

♡ Invest in quality stainless steel or nonstick pots and pans. This prevents scrubbing pots forever after meals. To keep food from sticking to stainless steel pots, heat the pot before you add oil or butter—food that gets stuck will come right off.

♡ Plan a soup or tomato sauce cooking marathon on a weekend, as a family or with friends or relatives. Make as many batches as you can and have containers at the ready, plus masking tape and markers to identify and date what you've prepared. Store batches in the freezer—they will make winter meals taste like summer ones.

♡ Freeze soups in individual-serving-size containers; thaw in a thermos for quick lunches.

♡ Cook with a "garbage bowl" on the counter. All the seeds, onion peels, and wrappers go right in there instead of all over the counter. Clean up is simply emptying the bowl!

♡ Use flexible cutting boards so you and your young sous chefs can easily scrape off into trash.

♡ Memorize the steps to your favorite concepts in this book so you can make a stir-fry or risotto without referring to the recipe.

♡ Cheat by writing the basic steps to your favorite concepts and taping them on the inside of a kitchen cabinet door over your prep area so you can peek when you forget.

10 time-saving products

product type	how to use it to save time
chicken, vegetable, fish broth	Create quick soups, pasta sauces, risotto, and stews
marinara sauce in a jar	Quick base for pasta recipes
frozen cooked clams or mussels	Thaw and add to sautéed onion and garlic, and add a bit of chicken broth. See the recipe for seasonal pasta in Day 23 "Eat Like a Roman."
frozen cooked seafood medley	Prepare as above; combine with fish broth and vegetables for a quick seafood soup, or put in miso soup; add to our quick marinara sauce recipe
frozen spinach or other chopped greens	Use to make spinach pie, quiche, spring omelet, or put in soups, stir-fries, or Italian pasta sauce
frozen peas and lima beans	Use in stews, risotto, rice, stir-fries, or swap out in other legume recipes
roasted peppers in a jar	Add to Italian pastas or salads
frozen fruit	Gets red and purple colors into your diet quickly; add to pancakes and pies when fresh berries aren't available
canned smoked oysters, trout, or other smoked fish	These add amazing flavor and substance to salads. You have to drain and rinse the oysters.
bread crumbs	You can make your own, but good, all-natural types are available. They can be a lifesaver when making the chicken tenders in this chapter.

♡ Invest in a dozen medium-size plastic bowls to use as mise en place bowls for prepped ingredients—if a child drops it, nothing breaks.

♡ Forget peeling vegetables, just scrub them well. Apart from puréed soups, you can leave the peels on root vegetables—peels are nutritious.

♡ Have kids peel potatoes or shuck corn over a plastic bag on the cutting board. When you're done, the bag goes right into the trash.

♡ Shop for perishable ingredients with both a recipe concept in mind and a back-up plan; if plans change, you switch gears and use the cauliflower for stir-fry rather than soup.

🕐 get started

Motivate your family to support you in making delicious, healthy meals more quickly:

♡ Use the international recipe concepts we provide for quick meals.

♡ Convene your family and outline the areas where you can use the most help; invite kids to choose which ones appeal to them.

♡ Explain that making mealtime a shared experience creates more time as a family.

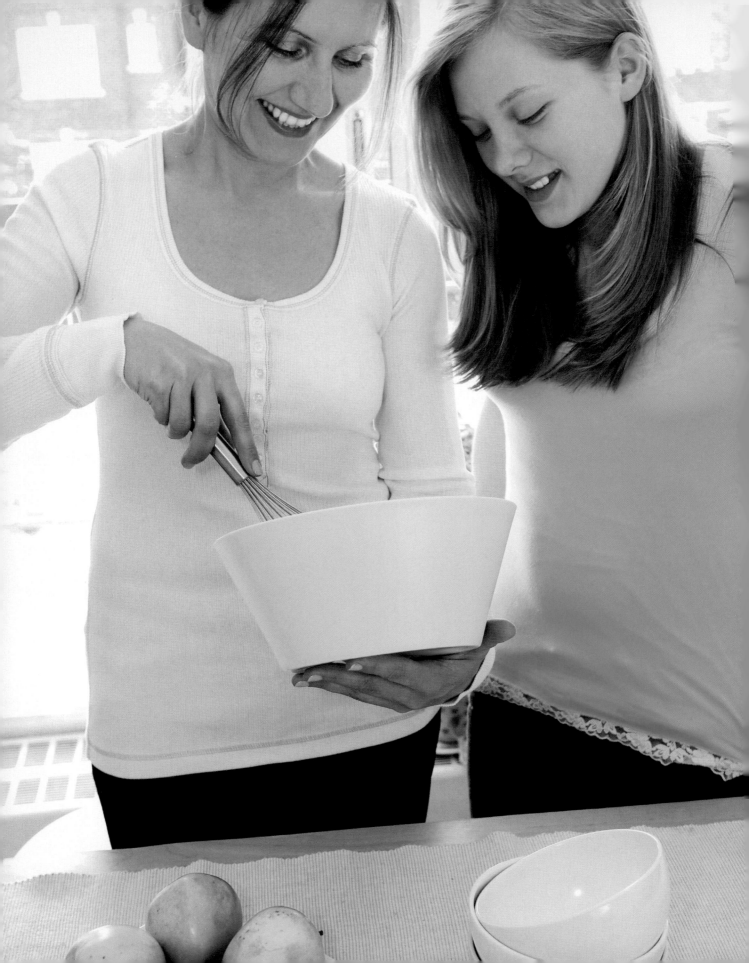

quick chicken tenders

An Italian chef in Umbria shared this quick kid-friendly chicken preparation with Lynn. She tried it at home with her boys, and it was met with cheers. It became a great default dinner solution.

1 pound (455 g) boneless chicken breasts

5 tablespoons (75 ml) extra-virgin olive oil, divided

⅓ to ½ cup (40 to 60 g) dried bread crumbs

Salt and freshly ground pepper

NOTE: *Children should use plastic or table knives for all child steps that require cutting or chopping.*

ADULT Cut the chicken breasts into 2-inch (5 cm)-long, narrow pieces that are bite-size (smaller if you have very young children). Place in a mixing bowl.

CHILD Help measure 2 tablespoons (30 ml) of the olive oil and all of the bread crumbs. Add to the chicken and mix thoroughly with a wooden spoon. Help season evenly with salt and pepper.

ADULT Heat a large stainless steel or cast iron skillet and add the remaining 3 tablespoons (45 ml) olive oil. Sauté the chicken for 6 to 8 minutes, turning as needed to brown evenly. Add more olive oil if it becomes too dry. Transfer to platter or individual plates to serve.

PREP TIME	COOK TIME	YIELD
5 minutes	5 to 8 minutes	4 servings

quick stuffed chicken breasts

When Lynn serves this dish to family or friends they think she's slaved all afternoon in the kitchen. The flavors are sophisticated and impressive, but in truth it's one of her time-saving showstoppers.

4 boneless chicken breasts, 4 to 6 ounces (115 to 170 g) each

Extra-virgin olive oil

Salt and pepper

3 ounces (85 g) pecorino, Gruyère, or other semimoist, semihard cheese

16 large fresh basil leaves

1 ounce (28 g) grana padano cheese

3 to 4 tablespoons (45 to 60 ml) extra-virgin olive oil

ADDITIONAL COOKING EQUIPMENT: Kitchen mallet, plastic wrap, toothpicks

NOTE: *Children should use plastic or table knives for all child steps that require cutting or chopping.*

ADULT & CHILD Spread the chicken breasts out on a cutting board and cover with plastic wrap. Pound each breast with the mallet until it becomes thinner and flatter. Remove the plastic wrap.

CHILD Drizzle some olive oil over each breast, then season with salt and pepper. Help grate semihard cheese. Spread the grated cheese evenly over the flattened breasts. Lay four basil leaves over the cheese on each breast, completely covering the cheese. Grate the grana padano over each breast.

ADULT & CHILD Starting at the narrowest end, roll up each breast to create a roulade, and secure with a toothpick. Moisten the outside of each with a bit more olive oil; season with additional salt and pepper.

ADULT Heat a large skillet or grill pan on high heat. Grease the pan with the 3 to 4 tablespoons (45 to 60 ml) olive oil. Cook the stuffed breasts until chicken is cooked throughout, about 12 minutes or more, depending on the size of the breasts. Check for doneness by cutting to check the meat is no longer pink before serving.

PREP TIME	COOK TIME	YIELD
5 minutes	12 to 15 minutes	4 servings

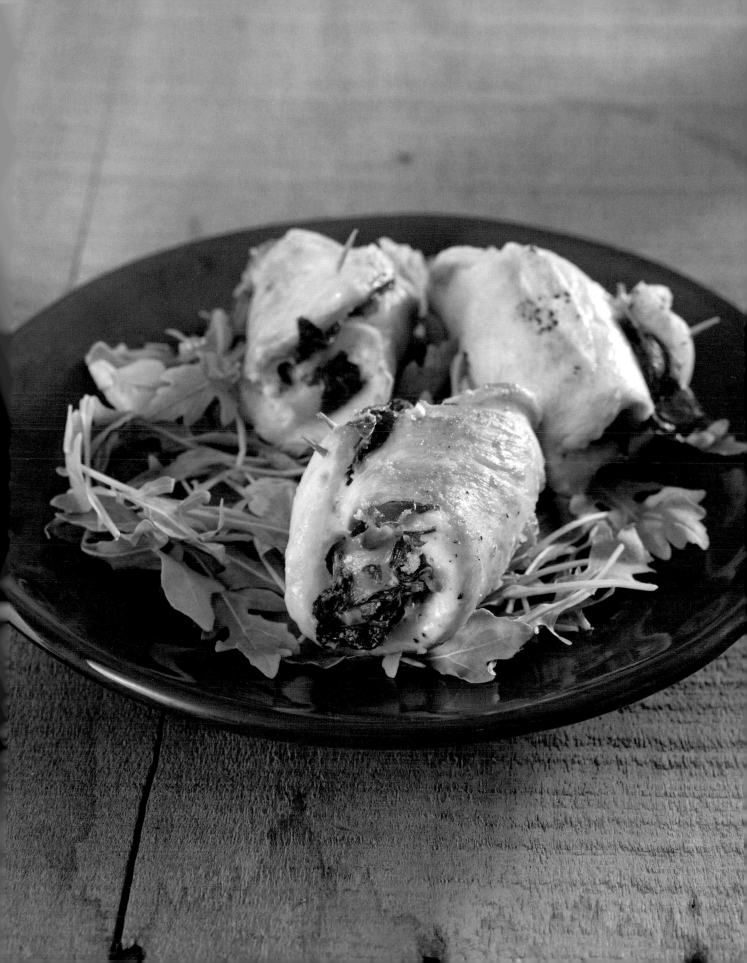

sweet pumpkin mash

The USDA dietary guidelines specifically recommend including dark-orange vegetables in your diet regularly. Using vegetables other than carrots can be challenging—until you try this recipe.

2 delicata squash, 1 acorn squash, or 1 sugar pumpkin

1 tablespoon (14 g) butter

1 tablespoon (15 g) packed brown sugar or maple syrup

Salt (optional)

NOTE: *Children should use plastic or table knives for all child steps that require cutting or chopping.*

ADULT Cut the squash in half (quarters if using acorn squash). Squash may be cooked in either the microwave or the oven. If using the oven, preheat to 400°F (200°C, or gas mark 6).

CHILD Help measure the butter and divide it into 4 equal pieces. Smear butter along the cut side of the each piece of squash.

ADULT Microwave on High until squash is very soft inside and butter is completely melted. Or if roasting, place the squash cut side down in a baking pan with ¼ inch (13 mm) water. Roast for about 30 minutes in the preheated oven. Cool.

ADULT & CHILD Use a spoon to scoop the cooked squash from the shell and into a mixing bowl.

ADULT & CHILD Mash the squash and season with the maple syrup or sugar. Season with a pinch of salt.

PREP TIME	**COOK TIME**	**YIELD**
5 minutes	12 minutes	4 servings

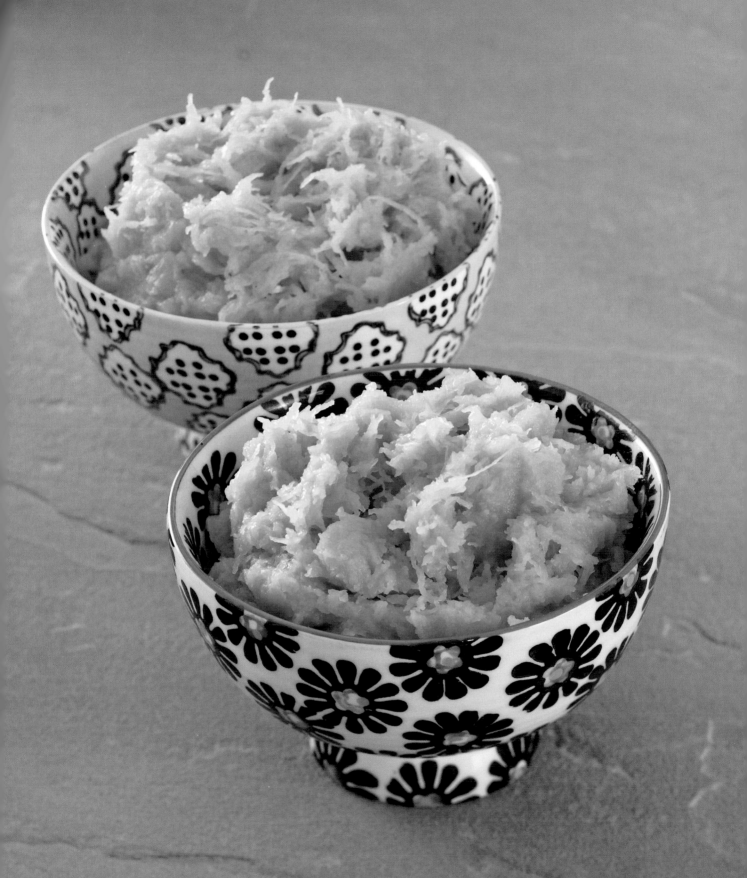

{DAY 25} Supercharge Breakfast

BREAKFAST IS ESSENTIAL to start the day off well nutritionally at any age. This is certainly true for children, whose growing minds and bodies need regular fueling. Going without food for long periods of time can cause physical, mental, and emotional problems in children and make it harder for them to concentrate in school. Skipping breakfast can also lead to weight gain because hungry children tend to nosh on high-calorie treats to hold them over until lunchtime.

The Academy of Nutrition and Dietetics reports that as many as 30 percent of children skip breakfast. Scientific studies show that aside from giving kids the energy they need to start the morning, a healthy breakfast can improve their cognitive function, memory, academic performance, and even their school attendance.

Teenagers are the major breakfast skippers. They stay up late and often get up before they are well rested. It's too early in the morning for them to be hungry, and they rush off to school without fueling up. By the time they do feel hungry, they're in the middle of a math class or science exam. Without the energy their brains need to function optimally, teens may perform more poorly than they would have if they'd eaten a healthy breakfast.

Missing breakfast is a bigger problem for kids than most parents realize. Because children's bodies are still forming, they have not developed the ability

> **MISSION FOR THE DAY**
>
> Surprise your family with an international breakfast.

to store nutrients during periods of fasting. Kids who skip breakfast may go without food for sixteen hours between dinner and their quick lunch the next day at school.

A healthy breakfast should provide a balance of complex carbohydrates and include fiber, protein, a little fat, and plenty of vitamins, minerals, and phytochemicals. Complex carbohydrates replenish blood glucose levels after fasting overnight. Glucose is the brain's main energy source, and it is necessary for concentration and alertness.

Many people skip breakfast to save time. But you don't have to spend a lot of time preparing or eating breakfast—the recipes in this book prove that.

sample healthy breakfast ideas from around the world

Want to break out of your humdrum breakfast routine? Take a tour around the world and let various cultures inspire you with their breakfasts.

Different cultures have different food customs and strategies that achieve the same nutritional needs. The rice in a Japanese breakfast, for instance, provides the carbohydrate energy that American cereal does. The fish provides protein, as does our bacon or ham, in addition to offering a healthy type of fat. Fish also contains calcium and other nutrients, especially when eaten with its soft bones. Soybean foods such as tofu supply protein, too.

Here are some of our favorite international breakfast strategies. They can give you ideas and inspiration for waking up your family's breakfast table:

- ♡ **peru:** Quinoa can be cooked like oatmeal. Here's another breakfast specialty: tamales made of corn dough wrapped around a traditional filling of cheese, meat, peanuts, chili, and vegetables.
- ♡ **singapore:** *Nasi lemak* is a rice dish made with coconut milk, fish, and fruit.
- ♡ **thailand:** Rice porridge is similar to the Chinese *congee*; stir raw egg into the hot liquid so it poaches.
- ♡ **china:** Dim sum breakfast offers an amazing variety of dishes and flavors. You can buy dim sum dumplings at the supermarket.
- ♡ **syria:** Sliced cucumber, Lebanese yogurt dip, Syrian cheese, olives, pita bread (perhaps toasted and served with cheese), or aromatically flavored za'atar bread are all traditional Syrian breakfast foods.

🕐 get started

If your family isn't used to eating breakfast, you may have to make some changes in their schedules to enjoy this important meal together:

- ♡ Adjust time schedules, and wake up children at least fifteen minutes earlier than usual to make sure they are awake enough to feel hungry.
- ♡ Prepare breakfast for children. Even if they are old enough to find or make their own breakfasts, they will have more incentive to eat if food is there waiting.

play food detective: how healthy are breakfast cereals?

Many children's cereals are really cookies in disguise. Typically they contain 40 to 50 percent sugars by weight. Assess these breakfast products to see how healthy they are:

- Look at the box designs to see how they motivate children to want the cereal.
- Compare the ingredient lists on various boxes. Which cereal has more added sugar?
- Count all the ingredients that are sugars. How close are they to the beginning of the ingredients list?
- Check ingredients for trans fats or hydrogenated oils or any other unnecessary oils.
- Check ingredients for unnecessary additives.
- Note that rolled oats contain only one ingredient: oats. When making oatmeal, you can add your own healthy sweetener, nuts, and fruits.
- With your "food detective" kids, discuss which cereal is healthier, and why.

- ♡ Pack breakfast to eat on the go—this is a good option, especially when children take a bus.
- ♡ Find out if your kids' school offers "Grab and Go" breakfast, which lets students get a bag breakfast to eat in class. This can be an option for hectic mornings. Ask what your child's school is serving and decide whether it's acceptable.
- ♡ Prepare waffle or pancake batter the night before and store in a sealed container. Then these breakfast favorites take only two minutes to make.
- ♡ Have plenty of fruit on hand, fresh and frozen. You can cut up strawberries, peaches, or other fruit into a bowl, then throw in some granola

A healthy breakfast should provide a balance of complex carbohydrates and include fiber, protein, a little fat, and plenty of vitamins, minerals, and phytochemicals.

and plain yogurt, and drizzle honey or agave syrup over it all for a nutritious breakfast in five minutes.

♡ A homemade smoothie that blends frozen or fresh berries, milk, and ice can be drunk quickly and contains lots of nutrients.

mercedes' story

During the year I lived in Japan, my Spanish siblings came to visit me, and I took them to a traditional, family-run bed and breakfast. I had already explained the different table manners in Japan and showed them how to use chopsticks. They found it amusing to sleep on the floor and bow to the hostess so many times. But their first breakfast prompted an unexpected surprise. "Soup, rice, and fish—for *breakfast*?" they asked.

The hostess explained they should scramble a raw egg in a small bowl, mix in some soy sauce, and pour the mixture on top of the bowl of rice. They then wrap the rice with a piece of nori (seaweed paper) and eat it, using their hands or chopsticks. My siblings had a memorable time, and we shared many laughs as they adjusted to these new breakfast foods.

rhubarb yogurt parfait

Rhubarb is underrated and often ignored, yet it provides vitamins and minerals, plus fiber. Make the compote in a large batch and freeze for the taste of spring in the dead of winter.

1 pound (455 g) rhubarb

⅓ cup (63 g) sugar or honey

½ cup (120 ml) water

3 cups (690 g) vanilla or plain low-fat yogurt

½ cup (75 g) fresh blueberries (optional)

NOTE: *Children should use plastic or table knives for all child steps that require cutting or chopping.*

ADULT & CHILD Cut the rhubarb into 2-inch (5 cm)-long pieces and place in a medium saucepan.

ADULT & CHILD Measure the sugar and add to the rhubarb.

ADULT & CHILD Measure the water and add to the saucepan. Stir to mix thoroughly.

ADULT Set saucepan over medium-high heat, and bring mixture to a boil. Lower heat and cook 5 to 10 minutes, or until the rhubarb breaks down and the mixture becomes runny, like a sauce. Remove from heat and cool.

ADULT & CHILD Layer ½ cup (115 g) yogurt into 6 serving cups or bowls (clear ones make a pretty presentation) with ¼ cup (75 g) rhubarb sauce. Top with blueberries and serve.

PREP TIME	COOK TIME	YIELD
10 minutes	10 minutes	6 servings

spring omelet

The delicate flavor of eggs and cauliflower and the fragrance of dill combine to make the dreaded green veggies more appealing and acceptable to children. You can change this recipe by using different types of greens, such as beet and turnip greens.

1 medium onion, or 2 leeks

1 tablespoon (15 ml) olive oil

2 tablespoons (28 g) butter, divided

5 ounces (140 g) chopped, cooked fresh or frozen greens

½ head, or 5 ounces (140 g) fresh or frozen cauliflower, cooked

4 eggs

½ teaspoon baking powder

1 teaspoon kosher or sea salt

½ teaspoon freshly ground black pepper

⅓ cup (21 g) fresh dill

Salt and freshly ground black pepper

NOTE: *Children should use plastic or table knives for all child steps that require cutting or chopping.*

tips

- Grow your own herbs and let the children snip them.

- Ask them what other veggies they might like to use in place of the cauliflower.

ADULT Chop the onion or clean and slice the leeks thinly.

ADULT Heat a medium skillet over medium heat and add the oil and 1 tablespoon (14 g) of the butter. Lower the heat, and cook the onions slowly, about 5 minutes, or until softened.

ADULT & CHILD Measure the cooked greens and set aside. Child can help measure and chop the cooked cauliflower.

ADULT & CHILD Crack the eggs on the edge of a medium mixing bowl; with two thumbs in the crack, separate the halves and drop the eggs into the bowl. Whisk eggs well.

CHILD Help measure the baking powder, salt, and pepper; add to egg mixture.

CHILD Chop the dill finely or snip with scissors.

CHILD Add the greens, cauliflower, and dill to the egg mixture. Mix well.

ADULT Add the onions to the egg mixture. Mix well.

ADULT Melt the remaining 1 tablespoon (14 g) butter in the skillet used to cook onions. Add the egg and veggie mixture and cook, covered, over medium heat, about 7 minutes, or until eggs are set. Season to taste with salt and pepper.

OPTIONAL COOKING METHOD: Preheat the oven to 400°F (200°C, or gas mark 6). Cook egg and veggie mixture until halfway set, then place skillet in the oven to finish cooking, about 5 minutes.

PREP TIME	COOK TIME	YIELD
15 minutes	20 minutes	4 to 6 servings

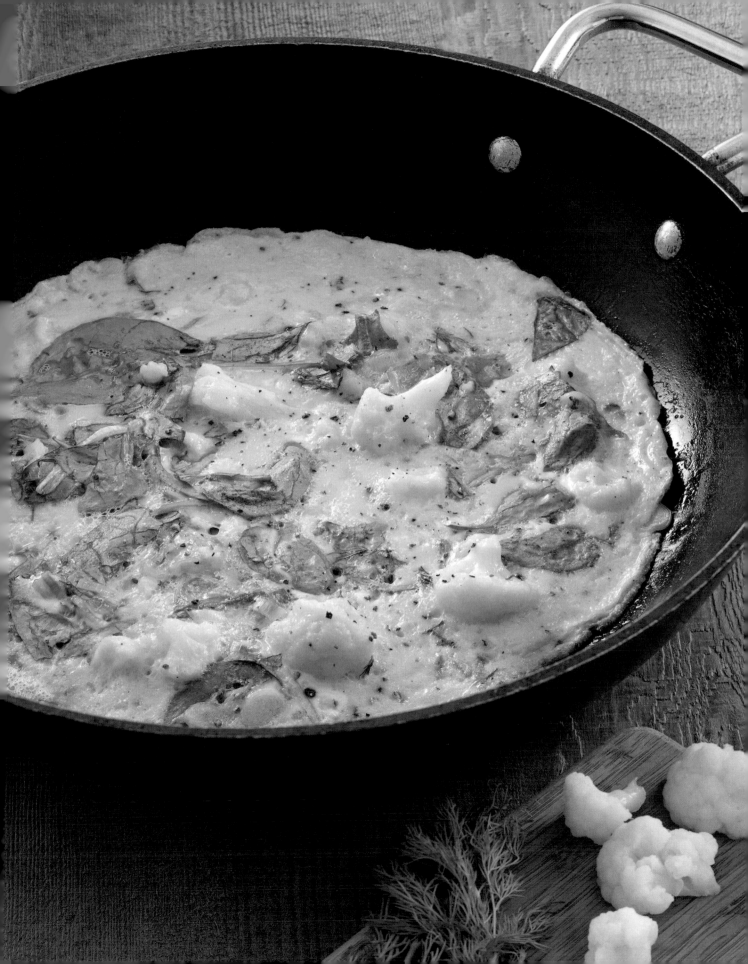

whole wheat pancakes

Whole-grain pancakes have more flavor and are more filling and nutritious than ones made with white flour. For nutritional benefits and great taste, top with real maple syrup.

1 tablespoon (15 ml) fresh lemon juice

2 cups (475 ml) milk

1 cup (100 g) unbleached flour

1 cup (130 g) whole wheat flour

2 tablespoons (26 g) sugar

2 teaspoons (9 g) baking powder

½ teaspoon baking soda

½ teaspoon salt

1 large egg

2 tablespoons (28 g) butter, melted

Oil or butter as needed, for oiling griddle

Fresh or frozen (thawed) blueberries

Real maple syrup

ADDITIONAL COOKING EQUIPMENT: Griddle (optional), or cast iron skillet or nonstick skillet

tip

Swap out ¼ cup (30g) of either flour with oat bran or other whole grain flour for variety.

CHILD Help measure the lemon juice and the milk. Add the juice to the milk and set aside.

ADULT & CHILD Measure flours, sugar, baking powder, baking soda, and salt into a large mixing bowl.

ADULT & CHILD Crack the egg on the edge of a small bowl; with two thumbs in the crack, separate the halves and drop the egg into the bowl. Beat the egg lightly. Add the beaten egg and the milk to dry ingredients. Mix everything together.

ADULT Heat and prepare griddle with oil or butter.

ADULT Ladle batter onto griddle to make 4 inch (10 cm) or smaller pancakes. Throw a handful of berries on top of each pancake.

ADULT Cook pancake on one side until brown, then flip to cook the other side.

ADULT Serve with real maple syrup.

PREP TIME	COOK TIME	YIELD
15 minutes	1 to 3 minutes each	16 to 18 pancakes, 4 inches (10 cm) wide each

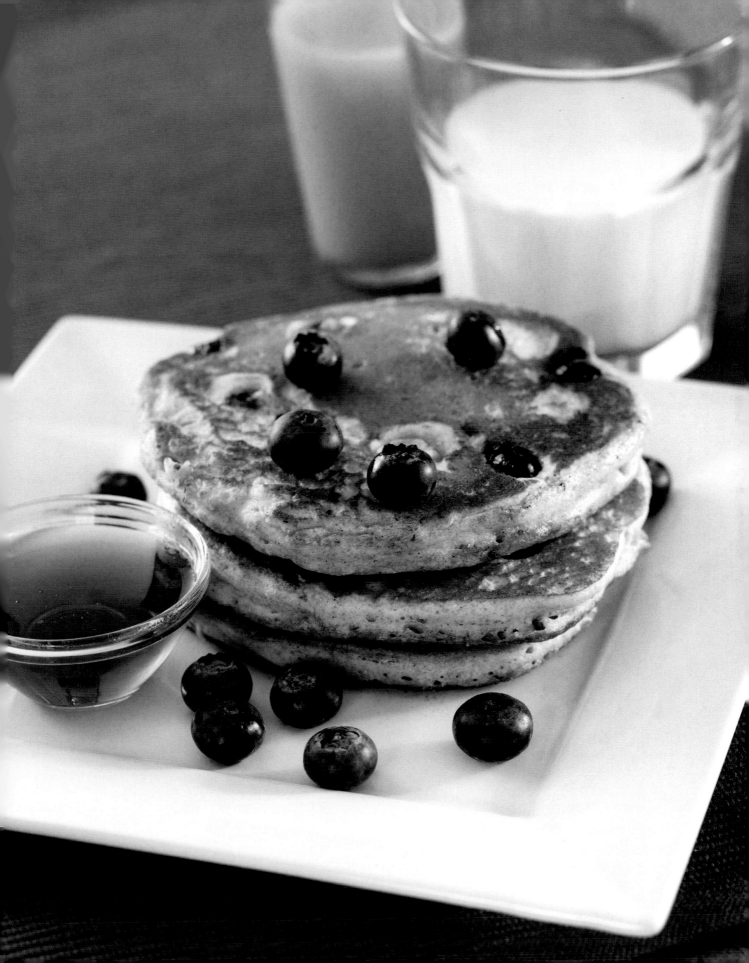

{DAY 26} Serve Healthy Portions

WOULD YOU MAKE a peanut butter sandwich for your child using five slices of bread? Serve him three baked potatoes for dinner? Make ten pieces of corn on the cob for single snack? Give her a glass of water with ten spoonfuls of sugar in it?

Yet as absurd as this may sound, we mindlessly do something similar when we give our children a New York-style bagel, McDonald's large fries, a large box of popcorn at the movies, or sugary sodas. And, of course, along with such insane portions come extra fat, sweeteners, and additives.

Eating out—which many of us do once or more a week—can be a real minefield when it comes to portions. Restaurants, food product manufacturers, and retailers work hard to convince us to take more than we need. This is especially true of restaurants that cater to families looking for value. Hence, our children are growing up not knowing what a normal, healthy serving size is. It's up to us, the parents, to show them by serving right-size portions and to teach them to analyze what they are offered when eating out.

mindless eating can lead to obesity

Thanks to researcher Brian Wansink, professor of consumer behavior at Cornell University and author of the best-selling book *Mindless Eating*, we are learning that many people are not "Master and Commander" of their food choices. Wansink's extensive research and behavioral experiments

MISSION FOR THE DAY

Be aware of how much you serve or are served.

demonstrate that people eat unconsciously when food is convenient, visible, and they are distracted. In one of his famous studies, a soup bowl was secretly refilled from under the table while people were eating and engaged in conversation. The study showed how diners mindlessly ate up to twice as much soup without noticing the extra food.

Food industry marketers, too, make large portions convenient and available when you are distracted, such as at a movie theater. As a result, many Americans develop unhealthy eating habits and don't listen to their bodies' signals that they're full. They end up consuming extra calories, many derived from sugars, highly refined carbs, and fats.

The addictive nature of sugary and salty foods, laden with flavor enhancers, makes it pleasurable to finish whatever size portion is served. But when we fill up on empty calories the body remains hungry for needed nutrients, which causes us to eat even more. This never-ending cycle can easily produce overweight and obese children and adults.

Lisa Young, author of *The Portion Teller Plan*, has tracked the astronomical growth in food portions, servings, and helpings in the United States during recent decades. She points to evidence that shows portion sizes are expanding, such as new dishwashers that accommodate larger dishware, and the increased size of pull-out drink holders in cars to accommodate mega-size beverages. Even cookbooks such as *The Joy of Cooking* have vastly increased serving sizes—a recipe that once made thirty brownies now suggests that the exact recipe yields only sixteen!

compare u.s. portions to those served in other countries

Traveling to other countries always opens our eyes. When we're in Europe or Asia, we see the food portions that used to be served in the United States a decade or two ago. In Paris you may be shocked if you order the famous *jambon beurre* sandwich on a fresh baguette with butter and sweet ham—it only has one small slice of ham in it! In Arab countries, coffee and mint tea are still served in tiny demitasse cups. In Japan, a bowl of rice for an adult is smaller than a child-size bowl in the United States. But hurry up—in many countries portion sizes are slowly following America's lead.

You don't need to hop on a plane to see what we're talking about, just visit some international restaurants with your children and observe: Japanese restaurants typically serve small portions. Spanish tapas restaurants serve meals on little plates. And Chinese dim sum consists of small dumplings and other delicacies in mini-portions.

get started

Here are some good strategies to help you and your family become more aware of healthy portion sizes:

- At home, eat on plates that are 10 inches (25 cm) in diameter or smaller; use 6- to 8-ounce (175 to 235 ml) glasses.
- Don't force children to finish everything.
- Cook whole foods. Studies show children are more likely to overeat sugary and salty convenience foods and sugary beverages.

mercedes' story

My French and Spanish visitors keep reminding me of the outrageous food portions I've come to accept in the United States. My refrigerator is a wonder to all—few countries sell such huge refrigerators to store so much food. Friends gape at my bowls, mugs, and plates that look as if they were made for giants. They are perplexed when Starbucks tells them "small" is not an option. One aunt asked if Americans have a gene mutation that allows them open their mouths like a crocodile to bite into enormous deli sandwiches or super-size burgers. And when food is served in a restaurant, they go speechless until I explain the concept of a doggy bag.

- Eat slowly, giving children (and yourself) time to feel the sense of fullness—it takes about twenty minutes for the brain to register satiety.
- Help kids learn to listen to their bodies. Discuss whether they feel satisfied, very full, or stuffed.
- At restaurants, eat family style. Order a few dishes, place them in the center of the table, and let each person use a small plate to choose his or her portion. Ask for a doggy bag for leftovers.
- When eating convenience meals, do not eat directly from a package or container. Transfer your take-out food to your real china and glasses. If you'll eat outside the home, bring lightweight plastic, reusable bowls and glasses of normal size with you and eat from them.
- Go to www.choosemyplate.gov for information about servings sizes according to ages.
- Discuss portion sizes with your children. Search online for portion distortion images and show your children how portion sizes of cookies, sodas, pizzas, spaghetti, french fries, and other foods and beverages have grown during the past forty years. They'll be amazed!

classic andalusian gazpacho

This traditional soup favorite requires no cooking and offers plenty of taste. It's also a good way to use up stale bread. It's the ideal way to celebrate the flavor of tomatoes at their peak in summer.

1 piece baguette, 2 inches (5 cm) long, crust discarded

2 cloves garlic

2 teaspoons (12 g) salt

2 tablespoons (30 ml) sherry vinegar, or to taste

1 teaspoon sugar

½ teaspoon ground cumin (optional)

2½ pounds (1.1 kg) ripe tomatoes

½ cup (120 ml) extra-virgin olive oil (preferably Spanish oil)

Finely chopped red and green bell peppers, for garnish

ADDITIONAL COOKING EQUIPMENT:
Food processor

NOTE: *Children should use plastic or table knives for all child steps that require cutting or chopping.*

ADULT & CHILD Soak the bread in water. Squeeze out excess water, and break up the bread into the bowl of a food processor.

ADULT Smash the garlic cloves with the flat side of a chef's knife to remove the peel. Slice the garlic.

CHILD Help chop the garlic and add to the food processor.

ADULT & CHILD Measure the salt, vinegar, sugar, and cumin. Add to the food processor.

ADULT & CHILD Adult cores and slices the tomatoes. Child helps add the tomato slices to the food processor.

ADULT & CHILD Measure the oil and add to the food processor. Process until smooth. Add a bit of water if a less thick consistency is preferred.

ADULT & CHILD Adult slices the bell peppers. Child helps dice the pepper slices for the garnish. Chill the soup before serving. Garnish with the diced peppers.

tips

- Try it with different varieties of heirloom tomatoes.

- Use Spanish olive oil for the most authentic flavor.

PREP TIME
15 minutes

YIELD
4 servings

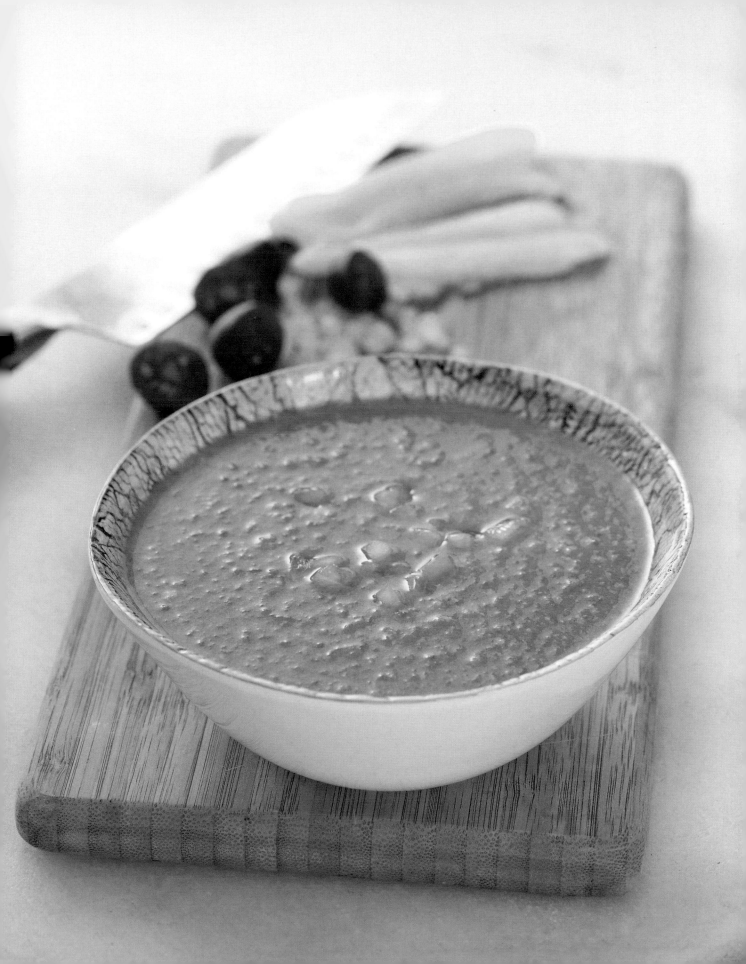

poached halibut with summer vegetables

This delicate, yet flavorful one-dish meal combines summer's beautiful colors and tastes.

½ cup (100 g) green beans or sugar snap peas

1 ear sweet corn, shucked

2 tomatoes

8 sprigs fresh dill

8 sprigs fresh flat-leaf Italian parsley

1 cup (235 ml) water

48 ounces (1.4 kg) halibut fillets

1 tablespoon (15 ml) extra-virgin olive oil

Kosher salt and freshly ground black pepper

NOTE: *Children should use plastic or table knives for all child steps that require cutting or chopping.*

ADULT & CHILD Cut the green beans or sugar snap peas into 1½-inch (3.8 cm) lengths.

ADULT Slice the bottom of the corn off the cob, and stand on the flat bottom. Slice the kernels off the ear of corn.

ADULT & CHILD Adult cores and slices the tomatoes. Child helps dice the tomato slices.

CHILD Remove the dill and parsley leaves from their stems and help chop them.

ADULT Heat the water in a small saucepan over medium heat until it simmers. Place the fillets in the water to poach.

CHILD Add the corn, tomatoes, dill, and parsley. Poach for about 6 minutes, or until fish is opaque and flaky.

ADULT Add the olive oil, and season the broth with salt and pepper to taste. Carefully transfer the fillets into shallow bowls and ladle broth and vegetables on top of the fillets.

PREP TIME	COOK TIME	YIELD
10 minutes	6 minutes	4 servings

{DAY 27} Hydrate Smart

UNTIL RECENTLY, people drank only water and beverages that came from plants and animals—fruit and vegetable juices, tea and coffee, and milk—plus some fermented beverages, such as beer, wine, and distilled spirits. But in recent decades, food manufacturers began tempting us with "magical" beverages, and they've built this into a billion-dollar-a-year industry. Now we drink not only to quench our thirst but to be smarter, cooler, sexier; to balance our electrolytes; to feel as successful as Olympic athletes; or to be superheroes.

skip the juice and eat fruit for better nutrition

Today shopping for beverages can be overwhelming. Our supermarkets carry fresh-squeezed, pasteurized or concentrate 100 percent fruit juice, 25 percent fruit juice, 10 percent fruit juice, and juicelike drinks that are little more than water with added fruit flavor. Or, if you prefer, you can choose from an array of "sports drinks" that supposedly rehydrate you better than plain old water, but can contain controversial and potentially harmful substances.

Our reaction to this development is simple and straightforward: We don't even go down those aisles in the supermarket. Our families drink water, tea, and sometimes 100 percent fruit juices, but generally mixed with water or carbonated water. Adults add coffee, wine or beer in moderation, and the occasional cocktail. What? No daily OJ? Isn't that un-American? Nope, it's just making a choice about the nutritional quality we want to achieve. We'd rather consume whole fruits that provide additional

> **MISSION FOR THE DAY**
>
> Drink and serve water as your only beverage today.

nutrition, such as fiber, than fructose-laden juices.

Beverage companies want us to see fruit juices as an essential part of a healthy diet. People who buy into that perception may let their children suck down so-called healthy juices as if they were drinking water. Check labels carefully when selecting fruit juices because what looks like 100 percent fruit juice may, in fact, be 100 percent vitamin C with water and sugars as the primary ingredients.

The next time you or someone in your family is thirsty, suggest nature's thirst quenchers: fresh fruits. Fruit is inherently a drink—with every bite you get an explosion of juice in your mouth. In summer, enjoy cold watermelon and other summer melons, coconut water, peaches, and plums. In fall, quench thirst with grapes, juicy pears, and apples. In winter, eat oranges, pomegranates, pineapples, and other tropical fruits.

say goodbye to sugary drinks that can cause health risks

According to a study published in the medical journal *Pediatrics*, the consumption of sugary beverages (sodas, sweetened iced tea, and other sugar-laden drinks) by children has risen dramatically in the last three decades. This increase is linked to excess weight gain, the risk of childhood obesity, many health problems including type 2 diabetes, poor nutrition, excess caffeine consumption, and tooth decay.

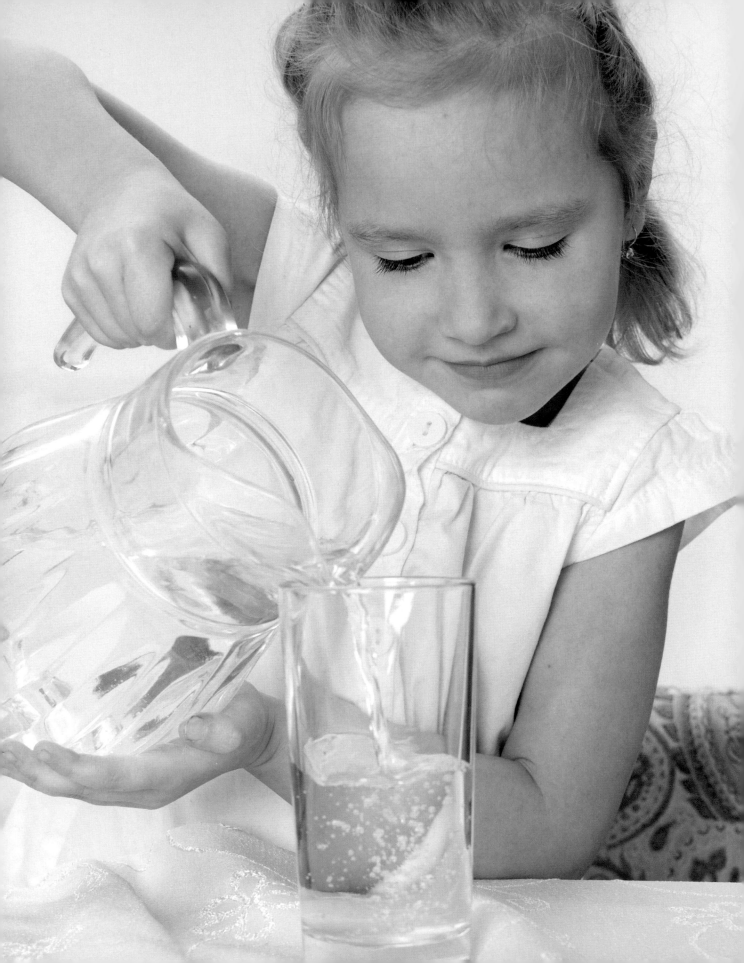

For adolescents, replacing healthy beverages, including milk, with sugary beverages is a significant problem. Between the ages of twelve and eighteen, young people require adequate calcium intake to fully mineralize their growing bones and to build adequate stores for their bodies' use throughout adulthood. To make matters worse, the high phosphoric acid content in cola beverages, in particular, can rob the bones of existing calcium, which may contribute to an increased possibility of bone fractures. By choosing sugary drinks, children may not only miss out on calcium, but also other crucial nutrients they need, such as riboflavin, vitamins A and C, and folate.

Sports drinks are cleverly marketed to children and adolescents as "healthy" alternatives to sodas. These were originally created as a dietary supplement for professional athletes, who undergo prolonged endurance training and whose rehydration is of extreme importance. But children who play or participate in organized sports don't expend that kind of energy. Kids can adequately rehydrate by simply eating a banana or plum along with drinking a cool glass of water or homemade lemonade. No need for the razzle-dazzle of specially designed drinks with extra sugar.

get started

Of course it will take some time to make the switch—you don't need to rush. Introduce these changes gradually and remember you're a role model. You may be surprised how quickly your family begins to follow your lead. Here are some ways to help you make the switch:

- ♡ "Drink" to your health with real, seasonal fruit.
- ♡ Offer children water and milk as primary drinks to quench their thirst.
- ♡ Add fresh mint, sliced strawberries, or a slice of orange, lemon, or lime to drinking water to make it festive and delicious.
- ♡ Add a handful of frozen mixed berries to a glass of water in summer to turn the water a pale pink; chill and enjoy the delicious fruit at the bottom of the glass.
- ♡ Drink homemade, freshly squeezed fruit juices as a treat.
- ♡ Drink 100 percent fruit juice (preferably not from concentrate) once in a while.
- ♡ Whether the juice is frozen concentrate, canned, bottled, or boxed, check the label to make sure it contains only 100 percent fruit juice.
- ♡ Always check the percentage of real fruit contained in a beverage. By law this information must be provided on the container, but it can be difficult to find if the fruit content is as low as 10 or 25 percent.
- ♡ Recognize and reject products with deceptive advertising such as "100 percent fruit blend," "100 percent vitamin C," or "fruit snack"—these appear to be healthier or more natural than they are.
- ♡ Avoid juice with added sugar.

In our "Teen Battle Chef" program, provided to students in inner city schools, we developed a "water challenge" to help students who drink far too much soda and sugary iced tea. The session begins with a discussion, as students drink water with lemon slices in it. After discussing the benefits of water and the harmful effects of soda, the students are challenged to switch from soda and other drinks to water—up to six glasses daily, for two weeks. The results? Most kids report they feel more energetic. Many of them are overweight, and they come to appreciate how drinking water before meals can help them feel more full, so that they don't overeat.

persian yogurt drink

Drinks that are a bit salty are popular in hot climates. This delicious yogurt drink is the perfect summer thirst quencher because it replaces the sodium that can be lost when you sweat.

8 ounces (225 g) plain yogurt, low-fat or regular

8 ounces (235 ml) water

½ teaspoon dried mint

Pinch of salt

Freshly ground black pepper

6 to 8 ice cubes (fewer if they are very large)

2 sprigs fresh mint

NOTE: *Children should use plastic or table knives for all child steps that require cutting or chopping.*

CHILD Help measure the yogurt and water into a pitcher. Mix well with a whisk.

ADULT & CHILD Measure the dried mint and salt and add to the pitcher. Season to taste with pepper. Mix well.

ADULT & CHILD Measure and add the ice.

CHILD Remove the leaves from the stems of the fresh mint. Roll the leaves between your fingers to release the aromatic oils.

ADULT Pour into glasses and garnish with the bruised mint.

danielle's watermelon cooler

Lynn's good friend and colleague Danielle O'Connell is a pilates and yoga instructor. She devised this drink for her clients. It's so tasty we had to share it here.

1 whole grapefruit

2 cups (100 g) watermelon chunks

8 ice cubes

1½ cups (355 ml) water

Pinch of sea salt

Agave nectar or raw honey

ADDITIONAL COOKING EQUIPMENT: Electric blender

NOTE: *Children should use plastic or table knives for all child steps that require cutting or chopping.*

CHILD Help peel the grapefruit. Keep the white membrane intact. Separate into segments.

ADULT & CHILD Dice the watermelon.

ADULT & CHILD Add the grapefruit, watermelon, ice cubes, and salt in the container of a blender. Process until smooth.

ADULT Sweeten to taste with agave nectar, processing as you adjust. Serve immediately.

PREP TIME 5 minutes | **YIELD** 2 glasses, 10 to 12 ounces each

PREP TIME 10 minutes | **YIELD** 3 glasses, 8 ounces (235 ml) each

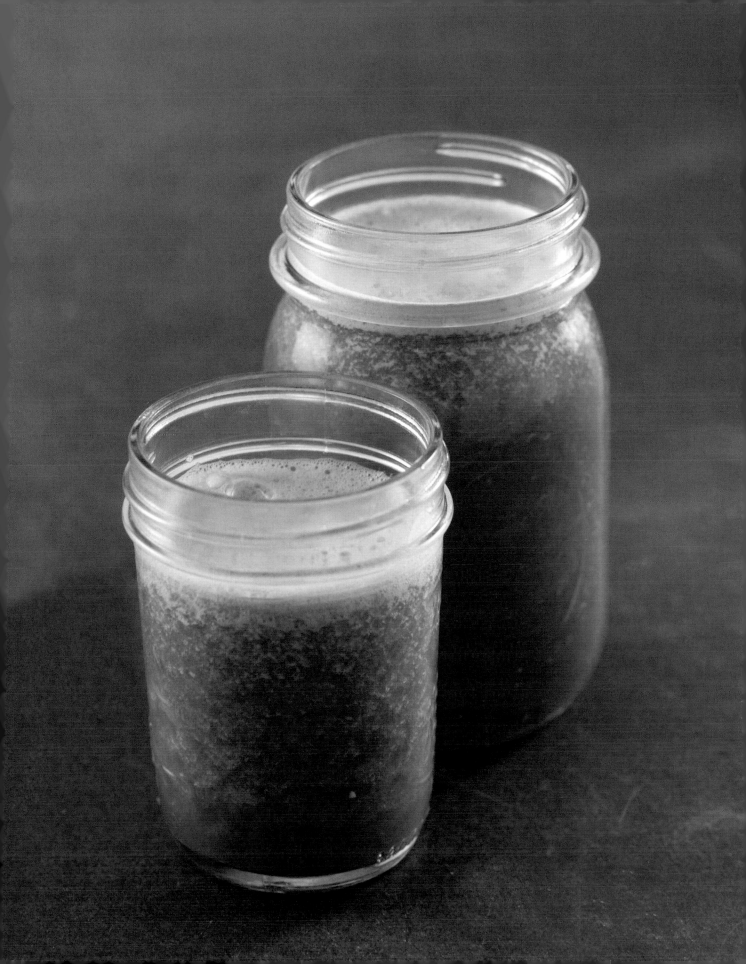

moroccan-style iced tea

This recipe transforms the most basic black tea into something festive and delicious. It's equally delicious hot or iced.

4 cups (946 ml) water

10 sprigs fresh mint

2 tablespoon (40 g) agave nectar

2 black tea bags (English Breakfast, Irish, nothing too aromatic)

ADULT Boil the water in a kettle over high heat.

CHILD Separate the mint leaves from the stems. Roll the leaves between your fingers to release the aromatic oils. Place in a teapot.

ADULT & CHILD Measure the agave and put it in teapot, then add the tea bags.

ADULT Measure ¼ cup (60 ml) of the boiling water and add to the teapot. Swirl the teapot for 1 to 2 minutes. Add the remaining 3½ cups (828 ml) boiling water. Let steep for 10 minutes.

ADULT Pour the tea into a pitcher and add ice. When chilled, serve with mint garnish.

PREP TIME
15 minutes

YIELD
4 glasses, 8 ounces (235 ml) each

PART 7

SHARE WHAT YOU'VE LEARNED WITH OTHERS

{DAY 28} Transform School Lunches

CHILDREN IN THE UNITED STATES eat about 180 meals at school each year. Do these meals reinforce the good messages that you're practicing at home? If you want to raise healthy eaters, you need to understand the difficult arena of the school lunch experience and what you can do to improve it.

understand the reality of lunchtime at your child's school

Can schools provide pleasant meals in a positive atmosphere where food is valued? You can't know unless you witness your child's lunch experience yourself. Observing school lunch can be eye opening, and you'll probably spot things you'd like to change.

Brief Lunch Breaks Don't Give Kids Time to Eat Healthy
Officially, children have thirty minutes for lunch, but that includes marching from the classroom to the cafeteria, waiting in line for food, waiting for a place to sit, cleaning up after eating, and lining up again. Actually, they have only about fifteen minutes to gobble their food! Rushing children through lunch doesn't transmit the message that their school values food. Many European schools break for two hours so children can enjoy a less rushed meal and have plenty of time to socialize and play.

MISSION FOR THE DAY
———
Volunteer at your children's school.

School Cafeterias Don't Offer a Pleasant Eating Environment
School cafeterias are often anything but inviting. Many are located in basements with bare walls and no natural light. The acoustics are terrible, especially if lunch tables are set up in the gym. When children socialize, they get noisy. In this hectic environment, it's hard to enjoy a pleasant meal.

A Healthy Lunch May Get Swapped for Junk Food
Cafeterias resemble Istanbul's Grand Bazaar. You sent your child to school with healthy food, but those baby carrots you packed in her lunch box are being traded for bigger currency—chips, cookies, and candy.

School Menus Don't Focus on Healthy Foods
Whether or not your children eat the school-prepared lunch, they are still exposed to the menu, which looks like the typical children's menu in any fast-food eatery: chicken nuggets, pizza, hamburgers, fries, tacos. No delicious and nutritious soup because kids could burn themselves while carrying it to the table.

mercedes' story

In PS321, my children's school in Brooklyn, New York, a science teacher with a vision, many volunteering parents, and a supportive principal successfully transformed the school's lunch experience.

The once-bare walls are now decorated with messages, photos, and art. Parents convinced SchoolFood Plus (the NYC Department of Education's healthy food initiative) to serve more vegetables and fruits, and they collaborated with the school nutritionist to change the lunchtime menu from hamburgers and chicken fingers to roasted chicken, a pasta salad bar, and vegetarian tacos.

A vegetable garden now grows in the schoolyard. Dedicated parents found grants to make this happen. Parents also help at lunchtime to improve the atmosphere and the food. They also got the vending machines removed from the school.

January is the month to celebrate "Green and Healthy." Teachers gear curricula to increase appreciation of whole foods. Parents cook with fresh ingredients in the classrooms. Children, excited by the momentum, ask their parents to put only healthy food in their lunch boxes. The month ends in a celebratory night with music and games.

Vending Machines Give Kids Easy Access to Sweets
You are lucky if your school doesn't have any vending machines. Even if children can't access the soft drinks, many vending machines are placed in prime locations for the convenience of the staff, where they flash advertisements to children.

resources to help you improve food programs at your child's school

- Learn about Alice Waters (www.edibleschoolyard. org), who achieved a revolution by planting a vegetable garden at the Martin Luther King Jr. Middle School in Berkeley, California, and creating a teaching kitchen.

- Want to organize a real school lunch transformation? Search online for "rethinking school lunch guide," a publication from the Center for Ecoliteracy (www.ecoliteracy.org), an organization that is active in school food reform and educates children about sustainable living.

- Check www.thelunchbox.org for recipes, strategies, and tutorial videos that have helped change school lunch programs across the United States.

- Find schools where improvements have happened and learn from them.

- Explore the feasibility of FamilyCook's "Jr./ Teen Battle Chef" (TBC) program (www. familycookproductions.com) at your child's middle or high school, or a partnership with an existing program for your elementary school (our partner HealthCorps runs TBC in 66 schools in the United States www.healthcorps. org). TBC student leaders learn to be "school food ambassadors" and support school food improvements while engaging the student body to have a voice in the changes.

- Become a member of your children's school's Wellness Council. If your school doesn't have one, assemble a group of concerned parents to use the federal mandate to start one, with the support of the school's principal.

- Write to your local and state representatives to demand more time for lunch.

- Go to Center for Science in the Public Interest (www.cspinet.org) to learn about school food policies. Support their national campaigns to get junk foods out of school.

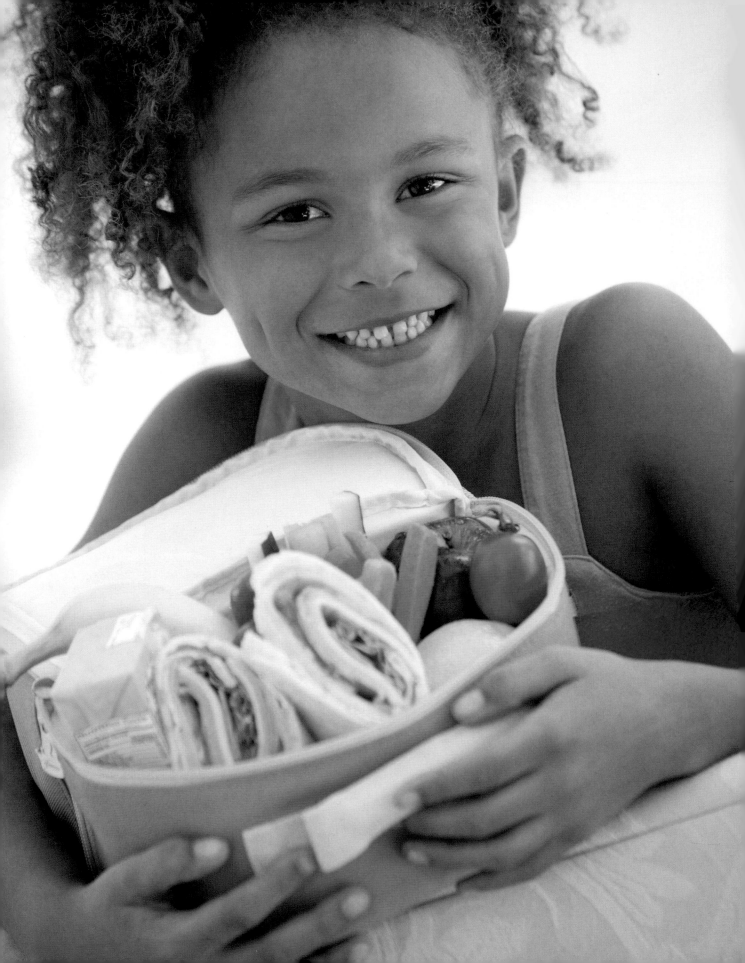

10 easy lunch box strategies you can try

How can you make school lunches fun for your children? These tips give you some colorful suggestions:

1 Japanese *bento* lunch boxes feature multi-compartment containers that invite kids to discover what's inside.

2 Thermoses let you send warm lunches with your kids to school. They'll enjoy the leftovers from the soups, stews, and pastas they helped make.

3 Surprise kids with this open-face sandwich: whole-grain bread with a filling of goat cheese; peanut or almond butter; or butter and mild cheddar. Top with edible petals from pansies, geraniums, or nasturtiums.

4 Choose some of the delicious salad concepts in this book and put the leftovers in mini-pitas.

5 Some lunch components are best packaged separately. Put chili in a thermos, wrap the bun separately, and put guacamole in a small container. Let your children assemble lunch and be the envy of their friends.

6 The recipe in this chapter for homemade energy bars is super popular with all ages.

7 Pack a cloth napkin of your child's favorite color in her lunch box.

8 Leave a written message inside your child's lunch box. He'll look forward to reading it every day.

9 Place a slip of paper that says "New Item: Thumbs Up/Down?" in your child's lunch box when you give her something new to try. Kids love to offer feedback.

10 Decorate his lunch box with stickers or pictures of his favorite cartoon or superhero characters. Leave a tiny toy in his lunch box as a "prize" when you introduce a new vegetable.

get started

Do you wish your child could be part of an Alice Waters Edible Schoolyard project, where children enjoy the produce they raise themselves at flower-decorated tables? Maybe it's time to advocate for change. Volunteer at your child's school and start transforming the way they do lunch:

♡ Check the wellness policy at your child's school. Ask the principal to ban certain foods from the lunch menu.

♡ Read a book about healthy food choices to your child's class.

♡ Help in the understaffed school kitchen during lunchtime.

♡ Cook a healthy, quick-and-easy recipe in your child's classroom.

♡ Help with fundraising so the school doesn't rely on money from junk food vending machines.

warm tuna wrap

Wrap sandwiches can be much more imaginative than what you'd find at your local deli. Forget all that tasteless lettuce and tomato, and try this version packed with flavor and nutrition.

½ of a 14-ounce (392 g) can white cannellini beans

1 can (5 ounces, or 140 g) tuna

1 clove garlic

1 tablespoon (15 ml) olive oil

Kosher salt and pepper

½ small turnip

1 small carrot

2 large radishes

2 springs fresh herbs (parsley, dill, cilantro, or combination), rinsed

2 slices lavash flatbread

4 ounces (115 g) feta cheese

½ lemon

NOTE: *Children should use plastic or table knives for all child steps that require cutting or chopping.*

ADULT Open the can of beans and drain in a colander and rinse well. Place half of the beans in a shallow bowl. Open the can of tuna and drain and rinse in the colander. Place tuna in a separate bowl. Smash the garlic cloves with the flat end of a knife to remove the peel. Slice the garlic.

CHILD Help chop the garlic slices finely.

ADULT Heat a dry small skillet over medium heat. Measure the olive oil and add to the skillet. Add the chopped garlic.

CHILD Mash the beans with a table fork.

ADULT Add the mashed beans to the skillet. Continue mashing the beans in the pan while mixing in with the garlic and oil. Cook on low heat about 2 minutes, or until heated through. Season to taste with salt and pepper. Remove from the heat.

ADULT Cut the turnip and carrot in half.

ADULT & CHILD Grate the turnip, carrot, and radishes using a box grater on a cutting board or in shallow bowl. Let children help by holding the end of the veggies while you hold their hands and help them go up and down once or twice. Older children can do this independently. Place each grated veggie in a separate small bowl.

CHILD Pluck the herb leaves from their stems. Help chop the leaves.

ADULT Warm one slice of flatbread in the microwave for 30 seconds (longer if necessary).

CHILD Place a slice of warmed flatbread on a cutting board. Spread about half the warm beans along the center of the flatbread. Layer the tuna and grated vegetables, and then crumble the cheese over all.

CHILD Squeeze some lemon juice over the sandwich.

ADULT Season lightly with salt and pepper. Roll the sandwich tightly. With a chef's knife, cut the wrap into bite-size pinwheels. Repeat with the second piece of flatbread.

PREP TIME	COOK TIME	YIELD
10 minutes	2 minutes	4 servings

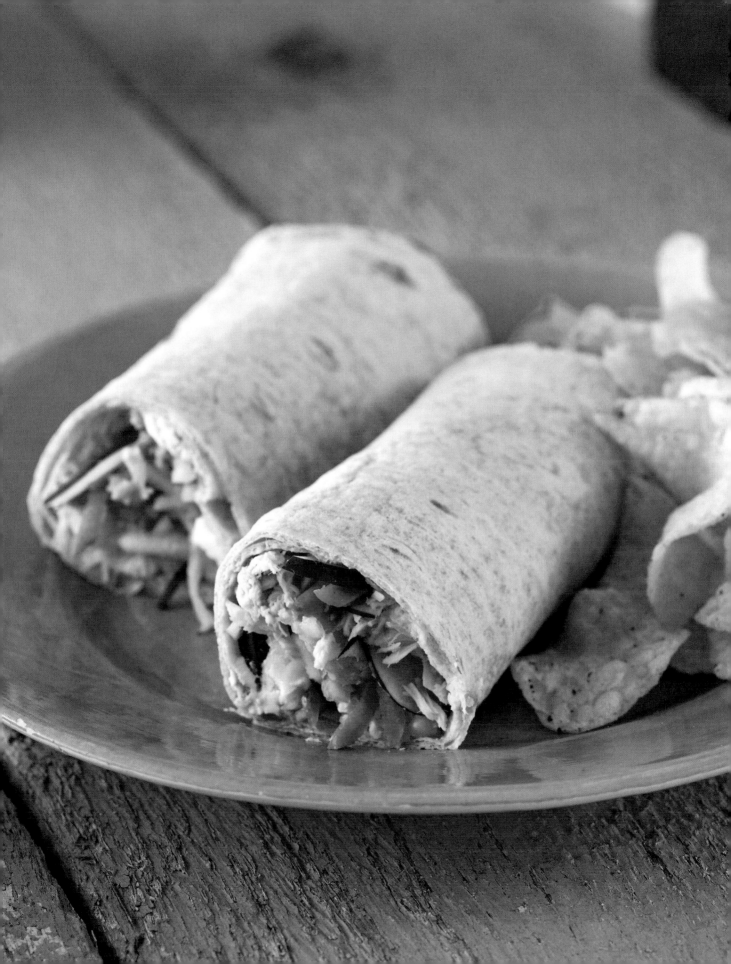

multigrain bars

This recipe is a more delicious and nutritious riff on the commonplace crispy rice treats.

¼ cup (36 g) sesame seeds

½ cup (110 g) chopped almonds

½ cup (75 g) chopped dried apricots, apples, or other dried fruit

½ cup (75 g) raisins or dried cranberries

2½ cups (53 g) puffed rice cereal

1¼ cups (100 g) rolled oats

½ cup (130 g) almond nut butter, smooth and preferably raw

½ cup (170 g) agave syrup

½ cup (170 g) liquid honey

1 teaspoon vanilla extract

ADDITIONAL COOKING EQUIPMENT:
8-inch (20 cm) square cake pan

ADULT Preheat oven to 300°F (150°C, or gas mark 2).

ADULT Place the sesame seeds and chopped almonds on a baking sheet lined with parchment paper. Toast in the preheated oven for 5 minutes.

CHILD Add almonds, sesame seeds, apricots, and raisins to a large mixing bowl. Mix well. Add the rice cereal and oats. Toss to combine.

ADULT In a large saucepan, whisk together the almond nut butter, agave, honey, and vanilla extract. Heat over medium-low heat for 5 minutes, or until mixture is just about to come to a boil. Remove from stove.

ADULT & CHILD Pour saucepan contents over the apricot-oat mixture, and mix well using large spoon.

CHILD Help grease the 8-inch (20 cm) square cake pan with light cooking oil or butter (nothing too flavorful). Press the mixture into the pan. Let stand for 30 minutes or until firm. Cut into 1-inch (2.5 cm) squares.

PREP TIME
15 minutes

COOK TIME
10 minutes

YIELD
About 3 dozen bars, 1-inch (2.5-cm) square each

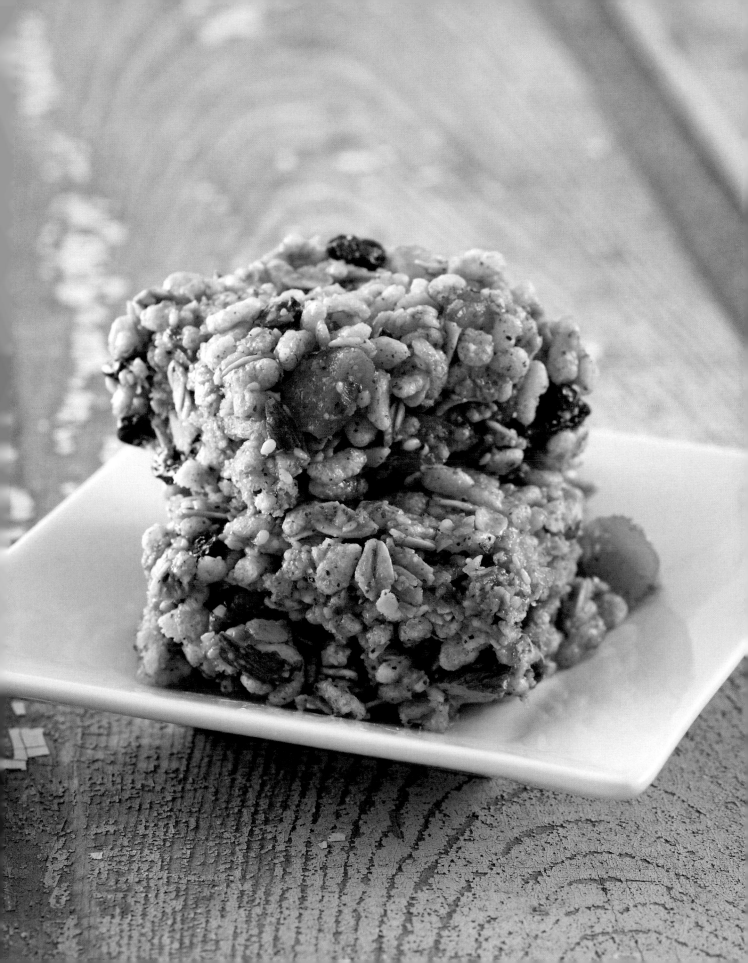

{DAY 29} Advocate for Your Family's Health

BY NOW, YOU AND YOUR FAMILY have transformed the way you prepare and eat meals, and your feel confident that you can develop a varied repertoire of delicious recipes that will make mealtime a special family time. But realistically, your family does not live in a cocoon, only eating what you serve and provide. The food landscape, as we all know, is much more complex. Once you venture into society, you are entering a minefield—an environment saturated with unhealthy food and beverages. You have no control over it. When you're away from home, you can find yourself in the midst of a battle where healthy choices come into conflict with the enticing convenience foods offered and promoted everywhere.

you can make a difference in the politics of food

Now that you have more knowledge and can distinguish what is healthy for your family to eat and what isn't, the next step becomes pretty clear. We need better governmental policies to regulate food production, packaging, and marketing so it's easier to make healthy choices.

MISSION FOR THE DAY

Select a topic within the realm of food politics that concerns you and read about it.

For more than eighteen years, through our program we have been helping families learn the skills they need to serve healthy foods. So it's exciting to see a food revolution around healthy choices brewing in the United States. The number of farmers' markets is on the rise, organic produce and products are filling up aisles in regular supermarkets, food advocacy groups are active in virtually every community, and the politics of food is a hot topic in mainstream media. It takes a village to go back to eating like our grandparents did.

As consumers demand and choose to buy quality foods, they send a strong message to the food industry and policy makers. As award-winning author and journalist Michael Pollan says, every day we are voting with our forks. But as parents, we also need to be vocal about the need for more regulations and policies that create equal access to healthy food at home and in our schools. Ask yourself these questions:

Both the Center for Science in the Public Interest and Environmental Working Group have plenty of active campaigns that need your support. These groups will also guide you if you want to write letters to your state representatives. They are both big supporters of improved school foods and limiting food marketing to children. Your advocacy will affect your children's future.

♡ Why is organic food and some local produce, dairy products, and meat more expensive than conventionally raised food, when the dangers of hormones, antibiotics, pesticides, and herbicides are well known? Why is it cheaper to buy junk food?

♡ Why does the federal government subsidize big agribusinesses while small local farms are going out of business?

♡ Why do coal-fired power plants continue to operate and contaminate our waterways and fish with mercury? Other industrial pollutants linger in many rivers and lakes.

♡ Why are junk food manufacturers allowed to market directly to children when research has shown this impedes healthy eating? A voluntary promise to reduce such marketing has recently been weakened as food companies are invoking their First Amendment rights to advertise to all audiences.

♡ Why can't I order a normal 8-ounce (235 ml) cup of my favorite drink? Or a normal-size portion of popcorn when I go to the movies?

♡ Why don't we have a right to know where *all* our food comes from—as citizen in many countries do—not just some of the produce, so we can choose to buy locally to support our communities?

♡ Why aren't the percentages of each ingredient contained in packaged food products listed on the labels?

♡ What percentages of added sugars are in the food or drinks we buy?

♡ Why isn't it made clear whether foods are made with genetically modified organisms?

⏱ get started

Learn from the experts. We know and have worked directly with the first two resources listed here. We utilize the third one to guide us specifically about produce purchases, to find out which contain unnecessary, unhealthy residues that we want to avoid. Visit these trusted resources' websites, learn about many more resources, and consider how you may wish to make your voice count:

♡ Dr. Marion Nestle (foodpolitics.com) of New York University has authored the books *Food Politics: How Food Industry Influences Nutrition and Health* and *What to Eat*. Both are eye-opening, well-researched introductions to how your food choices are manipulated and what you can do about it. Each day on her website, Dr. Nestle helps you understand up-to-the-minute controversies in food politics. She stirs up discussion, and the many comments from her readers are equally interesting.

♡ The Center for Science in the Public Interest (CSPI) (www.cspinet.org/) is a valuable, strong national advocacy organization that focuses on nutrition, health, food safety, and sound science. They're responsible for getting those Nutrition Fact labels put on all packaged foods in 1990, and later listing the amount of trans-fats. CSPI is always blowing the whistle on unsafe food or practices. At present it is involved in the area of food marketing directly to children. Don't miss their *Nutrition Action Healthletter*—it will keep you up to date with advocacy opportunities you can contribute to. And be sure to check out activities associated with CSPI's "Food Day" campaign so you can participate.

♡ HealthCorps, our national FamilyCook partner, which was founded by famed cardiologist, author, and television personality Dr. Mehmet Oz, has launched HealthCorps University (www. healthcorps.org). There, parents can mobilize to have health and wellness education and policies advanced in their school through training that HealthCorps provides to staff, administrators, and school food service workers. Through the U.S. national HealthCorps network, families can be part of national advocacy efforts for policy changes that will support health and wellness education in public schools.

♡ The Environmental Working Group (www .ewg.org/) publishes a "Shopper's Guide to Pesticides in Produce" and lists the famous "Dirty Dozen"—fruits and vegetables with the most pesticide residues—to help customers decide which are best to buy organic. It also lists the "Clean 15" you should consume if you can't afford to buy all organic or local produce.

♡ LocalHarvest.org connects you to local resources that are engaged in efforts to ensure everyone has access to healthy, fresh food. It tells you where the CSAs and food co-ops are and provides discussion forums.

♡ Find out if your local community or state has a food policy council. This can be a great group to advocate with around local food issues. Visit the Community Food Security Coalition's site (www.foodsecurity.org/FPC/) or WhyHunger.org and search keywords "food policy council" to find a food policy council near you.

This is only the tip of the iceberg for advocacy options. Marion Nestle has a long list of advocacy groups for every aspect of food matters on her website, under "FAQ." Take a look—there's a lot to be done!

{DAY 30} Make Food a Celebration

WHAT'S YOUR FAVORITE childhood memory of sharing food with your extended family? Was it at a table where dish after dish was presented with cheers? Was it the traditional birthday cake your grandmother made with pride and joy?

When we began this journey, we focused on taking pleasure in eating fresh, whole foods and teaching your children by example—making it a priority to prepare and enjoy family meals together. But why limit this experience to your immediate family?

sharing food with family and friends is fun

Regularly gathering with other people—friends and neighbors, as well as family—to enjoy delicious, healthy, home-cooked meals can provide great inspiration to stay on track. The Chinese gather around dim sum on Sundays. In Spain, weekends are for enjoying a festive paella with all the family. When Lynn was a little girl, she and most of her friends ate dinner at their grandparents' homes on Sundays. Today, many Italian-Americans preserve the traditions of Sunday lunch or dinner as a family.

As food historians note, special dishes give meaning to various cultures' celebratory traditions. When people raised their own food, entire celebrations developed around rituals to give thanks and show appreciation for an animal's slaughter and for a harvest (such as our Thanksgiving). Persian New Year Soup (see Day 11), for instance, is a key component of the Persian New Year celebration,

MISSION FOR THE DAY

Invite your friends over for dinner.

Norooz. What are your family's traditional celebratory dishes?

Today, the ritual of preparing special foods to ring in the New Year or celebrate Thanksgiving is losing ground to the popularity of dining out. Two decades ago, few stores and restaurants stayed open on holidays. Now they make a big point of marketing their holiday menus, prix fixe meals, and festive touches for such occasions. Even casual entertaining can seem like too much work when countless new restaurants are promoting their specials.

In this last chapter, we are not going to stray from our message of celebrating by cooking simply and meaningfully. Instead, we're going to expand that message to include people beyond your immediate household.

Entertaining friends frequently and with minimal fuss sends a valuable message to our children: food and family and friends go together, and eating this way is great fun.

Now that you've learned to cook dishes from around the world, why not share this adventure with others? If you don't have extended family nearby, invite friends, preferably with children who are close in age to your own so they can play together and parents can relax. You can take turns sharing meals with a small group of friends or just one other

mercedes' story

Each summer in Spain, our family meals included all ages, and everyone sat together, telling stories, many of which involved food. My children were like sponges soaking up the Spanish culture. When we returned to New York, I did my best to carry on the tradition.

On the weekends, we regularly invited friends to bring their children, and we'd cook. Nothing was especially elaborate, and I did not stay up until the wee hours the night before. We approached it casually, and our friends helped us cook. The children sat with us, or if there were too many of them to accommodate, at their own table.

As in Spain, we all ate the same food. Sometimes it was a traditional Spanish dish, but often it was a new dish that our friends wanted to share or that I wanted to try. My children loved the festive nature of these weekend meals and did not miss the chicken nuggets and mac 'n' cheese on kids' menus in most restaurants.

family. Or plan a cooking party. Invite friends to come and help you assemble an agreed-upon menu. Whichever style you choose, the tips that follow will make things easier and really fun! Just don't make it so special you only do it on rare occasions. Rather, do it frequently—let your children associate food and meals with a party at your house.

easy steps for entertaining at home

When you are entertaining at home, be sure to get everyone involved. Bring children into the entire celebration, from letting them help choose a theme to decorating for the occasion to preparing the meal and cleaning up. Here are some suggestions we've enjoyed, and hope you will, too.

Choose a Theme and Create Ambiance

Let everyone take part in choosing one of the cultures and recipes in this book. Find ways to add to the atmosphere:

- ♡ Download music from that culture to listen to while you cook and during the meal.
- ♡ Find a family film that matches the theme. This can make an evening festive even when you don't have guests.

Set the Dining Table Attractively

Welcome guests with a festive table set with candles, flowers, and decorative napkins:

- ♡ Have kids tie colored ribbons around the napkins, instead of using napkin rings.
- ♡ Use potted flowers or herbs in an attractive container for a centerpiece.
- ♡ Place numerous votive candles on the table. If you don't have holders, set three candles on a saucer and position two or three saucers on the table.
- ♡ Spread colorful fabric, a placemat, or even pillowcases folded to look like a runner under the centerpiece to add festive color.
- ♡ Let kids design and make place cards for everyone.

Serve Healthy Hors D'oeuvres

Choose and arrange a selection of these items and have them ready on platters or trays when your guests arrive:

- ♡ Serve two or three different types of artisanal cheeses.
- ♡ Add a nice jam or honey that goes with cheese—ask the cheese monger for ideas.

♡ Have kids arrange fresh fruits next to the cheese—grape clusters, sliced seasonal fruits, or dried fruits.

♡ Serve some boiled edamame.

♡ Let children set out a selection of nuts.

♡ Serve a few different patés or charcuteries.

Prepare a Simple Menu

Keep it to three courses—a salad or soup starter, followed by a main course, and a simple fruit dessert:

♡ Don't worry if your starter doesn't match your main theme. You can give your soup or salad a hint of your chosen cultural theme by using spices typical of that culture.

♡ Ditto with dessert. Plan your dessert around a fruit that would be typically enjoyed in that culture. Get kids to research online if you're not sure.

♡ Devise a festive juice-based beverage for the children, or add citrus rings to sparkling water to make it like a special cocktail. Colorful cups and straws will also be hits.

Serve the Meal Family Style

Keep it simple, and let everyone serve themselves:

♡ Serve the main course family style. It's festive to have a big platter or bowl on the table, from which everyone can take what they want, and it saves you the work of arranging each plate.

♡ Use a sideboard or island to place the main course platter(s), and everyone can fill their plates. Beverage refills can be placed here as well.

Simplify Clean Up

Make clean up easy by preparing for it in advance:

♡ Have kids empty the dishwasher before the guests come.

♡ Clean as you go; when guests arrive you should only have out food in pots or bowls, a clean counter, and a cutting board.

♡ Children can empty the trash before guests arrive.

♡ Ask everyone to clear his or her own place, rinse plates and silverware, and put them in the dishwasher.

♡ Let kids help put leftovers in storage containers and place them in the fridge immediately after dinner. This should leave you with only pots, platters, and bowls to clean. If you have a teenager, cleaning these the next day could be his or her task.

By now, if you've worked through this book sequentially, or at least thoroughly, you are the envy of your friends and extended family. You know how to feed your whole family in a healthier way. You can whip up a tasty meal from scratch using what you have on hand in your pantry, fridge, and freezer—you can even handle last-minute guests with the shrug of a shoulder. Armed with your chef's knife, you make quick work of fresh farmers' market produce and your children love munching raw veggies.

Are you a neurotic health nut? Absolutely not. You have made an important commitment to whole foods, home cooking, and sit-down meals. You've resurrected these values from your ancestors, and maybe you celebrate family or ethnic pride in the recipes you serve. You've made a huge shift. Now go enjoy your favorite healthy snack and give yourself a big pat on the back!

Acknowledgments

This book project is the result of the fortuitous coming together of our years of collaborating at FamilyCook and our editor at Fair Winds Press, Jill Alexander. From there many talented people on the Fair Winds team have proved to share our vision to inspire families around healthful meals cooked at home: Skye Alexander, Andrea Rud, Heather Godin, John Gettings, Debbie Berne, Glenn Scott, and Alisa Neely.

Throughout our writing and reviewing process we extend our thanks to those on whom we have relied heavily for recipe testing and/or editorial feedback and other support: Rebecca Zweig, Thalia Patillo, Kamen Asher, Lily Mercer, and to friends and colleagues for support and assistance: Chris Cook, Jimmy Lenner Jr., my son, Alex Fathalla, and dear friend Linda C. Levy.

L.F.—Because this book contains the essence of over seventeen years of professional focus around family togetherness and healthy eating, I owe my deepest gratitude to my immediate family: my sons Alex and Stephan, my mother EIleen Staats, her mother, my Nana, Ann Rudison, who taught me so much about food being inextricable from family, and my sister Lori Anderson. Other colleagues, friends, and those who have served on our FamilyCook team or supported our work along the way are too numerous to mention by name, but thanks especially to Dr. Antonia Demas, Michelle Feeney, Hazel Witte, Mary and Stephen Saint-Onge, Loren Talbot, Hilary Baum, Kerry Truman, Dr. Judith Wiley-Rosett, Dr. Deirdra Chester, Danielle O'Connell, Marion Nestle, Doug Anderson, Khahlidra Levister, Michelle Paige-Paterson, Janice Adams-King, and Dr Sharon Akabas.

And because it "takes a village," many thanks to our most committed and longtime collaborators: Michelle Bouchard and her stellar team at HealthCorps and founder Dr. Mehmet Oz, YMCA of Greater Rochester, Bob Lewis, Montefiore School Health Program, Northern Spy Food Company, Brooklyn Salsa Company, Jimmy Carbone, Teacher's College, Columbia's Institute of Human Nutrition, Albert Einstein College of Medicine, 15 Foundation, Urban Assembly Schools, Boys Club of New York, American Heart Association, EmblemHealth, Meyer Corporation, Share Our Strength, Chipotle Mexican Grill, Whole Foods Markets, 4Food, and OXO.

M.S.—Thanks to my husband for making mealtimes always special; to my daughter, Sofia, for cooking on those days I had deadlines, and to my son, David, for trying so hard to eat garlic and onions. Special thanks to my mother for cooking every single day of my childhood and inspiring me to prioritize home cooking for my children. Thanks also to my aunt Jennefer Hishbergh for her generous time reviewing the book and to Anne Kleinman and Vicki Hacken for their support during the early stages of this book project.

Finally, our deep appreciation and thanks to the many thousands of parents and children and program coordinators with whom we've worked in public elementary and high schools, WIC centers, and preschools, after school programs and more over seventeen years.

About the Authors

Lynn Fredericks is the founder of FamilyCook Productions (www.familycookproductions.com) and an award-winning pioneer in the field of obesity prevention and family nutrition. Since 1995, the educational efforts under FamilyCook Productions have reached over 100,000 families. A leading advocate for hands-on food/nutrition education for all, she is a popular lecturer, television personality, and cooking demonstrator. Together with her FamilyCook Productions' team of dieticians, chefs, and youth development professionals, Ms. Fredericks has developed research-based food and nutrition programs for state and local health departments, nonprofits, and companies. In partnership with HealthCorps, founded by renowned cardiologist, author and television personality Dr. Mehmet Oz and his wife Lisa, her Teen Battle Chef program has grown to over 100 schools across the U.S., empowering youth to make measurable improvements in their eating habits and "stir up change" in their communities by sharing their cooking skills and teaching others. In addition, Ms. Fredericks and FamilyCook programs have been featured on such national television shows as NBC's Today, Cooking Live, and the Food Network's Chopped, as well as numerous local radio and television programs around the United States. She lives in New York City.

Mercedes Sanchez has been Director of Nutrition Education for FamilyCook Productions for more than ten years. A registered dietician, Ms, Sanchez specializes in pediatrics and family nutrition. She grounds the FamilyCook nutritional messages, educational materials, curriculum and approach in the values that support the social and educational aspects of family meals. She holds a master's in clinical nutrition from NYU and has served as a dietician for the pediatric department of Methodist Hospital, in Brooklyn, New York. Ms. Sanchez is a true global citizen, having lived in Spain, Japan, USA and France. Her article on the value of a multicultural approach to teach children about nutrition was published in an Italian journal on taste, Questione di Gusti, in 2006. Ms. Sanchez's appreciation for celebratory meals prepared and enjoyed with family and friends hails back to her robust childhood as the youngest of nine siblings in Madrid, Spain. A mother of two young children herself, Sofia, 14. and David, 8, she understands very well the challenges that working parents face to navigate a social environment that tempts adults and children alike to take the easy way out and buy fast or prepared foods. She currently resides outside Paris with her husband and children.

Index